To Tim Enjoy
to Help /
Andy Curls.

AA GEMS

MEDITATIONS ON ALCOHOLISM
AND RECOVERY

AA GEMS

MEDITATIONS ON ALCOHOLISM AND RECOVERY

By Andy C

Copyright © 2019 Andy C

All rights reserved. No part of this publication may be
reproduced, stored in retrieval system, copied in any form or
by any means, electronic, mechanical, photocopying, recording
or otherwise transmitted without written permission from the
publisher. You must not circulate this book in any format.

ISBN: 9781999240707

Table of Contents

Preface	xi
Note on Authorship and Anonymity	xii
Introduction	xiii

LONGER-TERM AA — 17

Introduction	17
Right and Wrong Questions	19
Good habits — Bad habits	20
Checking out your Serenity	22
Separating the men from the boys	24
Static Build-Up in My Head	26
Atheist spirituality	28
When is God in your life?	30
Michaelangelo or Mickey Mouse	32
Putting boundaries on recovery	34

SERENITY AND GROWTH — 37

Introduction	37
Emotional Sobriety	38
Hallmark of Fear	41
Pre-flight checklist	43
Host to God or Slave to My Ego, Part 1	45
Host to God or Slave to My Ego, Part 2	46
Rule of Three Ups	48
Find Serenity — Pray for the Son of a Bitch	50
Into Actions	52
If You Spot It, You Got It	54
Spiritual Naps	55
Push My Buttons — See What You Get	56
Morning Meditation	58
Being Where I Am	60

How do I look to God?   62
Giving or Getting   64

STEPS   65

Introduction   65
12 Steps to Build a House   67
Reawakenings and Second Awakenings   69
Awakenings or Awakening   70
A Great Article by Bill W from the June 1958 Grapevine   72
Spiritual Maintenance   75
It is Only Coincidental   77
What Should I Expect from God?   78
A Gateway Step   80
The Tarzan Effect   82
Practicing Step 11, by Bill Wilson   84
Getting Out of the Rooms   87
Mental Real Estate   89

SELF-WILL / EGO   91

Introduction   91
Came Hard and Remained Firm   93
Good Start to the Day   95
Do I Need an Audience?   97
Anger and Perfectionism   98
Unconscious Contact with God   100
Upsettable with Myself   101
Dry Spells   103
The Safe Cracker and the Businessman   104
A Sidewise Glance   106

INVENTORIES AND BEYOND   107

Introduction   107

Ashamed   109
The Exact Nature   110
Not the Same Old, Same Old   111
Patterns Revealed, Secrets Denied   113
Inventories Get Easier   115
Inventory taking   117
Fearful and Shameful Inventory   119
Deeper Over Time   121
Habits of Meditation   123
Four Columns of Insight   125
Fifth Step, Redux   127

ACRONYMS AND WORD PLAY   129

Introduction   129
ID the ID   131
Alcoholic Thinking? GIGO?   132
The Meaning of Resentment   134
A2   136
The last stop   138
ISM Incredibly Short and Shallow Memory   140
Abandon or Surrender   141
Because You are NUTS, You are Nuts.   142
Non-Sequiters — Even When You Don't Want To   143
Now Here — Nowhere   145
EGO — Edging God Out   146
Sobriety is not Circumstantial   148

A PARTING GEM   149

Unconditional Love   149

Bibliography   151
Books that have meant a lot to me   153
Biography   157

Preface

Where did these GEMS come from?

When I am listening to fellow alcoholics share at Meetings, I take notes. Not transcriptions, just notes of things that catch my attention. By jotting a reminder, I can later recall the thought.

One night, my sponsor asked me, "What do you do with your notes?"

"I keep them and reread them, often the next morning during my morning quiet time," I replied. "They bring to mind the wisdom and humour that I heard. I meditate on the comments and see the insights that I missed. I feel grateful all over again… then I throw them away."

"You should write your thoughts down and share them," he said, "You might have some fun and it might do some good."

So I started writing my meditations. In the beginning, I only shared them with my sponsees, who passed the notes to their sponsees, and then others in the Program. A couple of the recipients, involved in treatment centres with newsletters, reposted them in their newsletters and websites. They seemed to attract attention, so I started a website — the4thdimension.ca — and posted them online.

One day I thought, "Maybe a book is a good idea."

So, these GEMS are my meditations. Drawn from Meetings, observations, readings, these notes from my life are GEMS I have discovered while trudging my road to Happy Destiny.

I hope that you enjoy reading them as much as I did writing them.

Note on Authorship and Anonymity

In the Program of AA, we are anonymous, but privately, we can be open.

If you want to contact me, you can send me an email at the address below, and I will strive to get back to you.

andyc@the4thdimension.ca

Introduction

I had arrived at my Home Group for our AA Meeting. A fellow sat down across the room. I didn't recognize him. So, I walked over. "Are you new?" I asked.

"No," he said, "I have been around for a long time, but it's been a long time since I've been to a Meeting."

"Welcome, good to see you – it took a lot of courage to walk in here tonight, and it is great to have you with us. We have herbal tea in the kitchen; we decided to forego coffee late at night."

"Thanks," said he. "I think I'll pass, but thanks anyway."

He seemed out of sorts. I asked my favourite question, "What Step are you working on?"

"Oh, I did the Steps a long time ago."

"Ahhhh, then you must be on Step One."

He laughed. And so began a new sponsee relationship.

Over the years, God has blessed me with the association of many Long-Timers who have come back. Some after drinking, and others, like my new friend, had not gone back to drinking but had drifted away from the Rooms. They had to break through the doubt and shame and come back to the Rooms.

Long-Timers have years. Old-Timers have wisdom. I have acquired small amounts of wisdom from the passage of time. But more has been acquired through periods of Program dryness, periods of spiritual drought. Fortunately, every time I have walked through the deserts of dryness, I have come out the other side still sober. Others have not; they lost track of the Program and spiritual growth. Many have succumbed to John Barleycorn, our cunning, baffling, and powerful foe.

My experience and observation of spiritual droughts and Program dry spells lead me to some tentative conclusions about these phenomena. There seem to be categories of types and causes.

The most common are drifters. They drift away from the Program. I have drifted in my Program. No crisis, just boredom and apathy. I was a young lawyer paying for parking one day. As the parking lot attendant gave me my change from his kiosk, I thought "It would be nice to be a parking lot attendant." I had lost any sense of meaning and purpose. I had confused serenity with boredom. I had lost energy for life and the Program. I did not reconnect till one day I asked a fellow in the Program if he would sponsor me. That started a walk back to God. I rediscovered purpose.

Another problem is success. Sometimes we call it complacency. AA's sober up, become successful and develop a growing sense of independence. In my own case, I was succeeding and making money. My reputation as a good citizen was growing. I began to think that my sobriety was all because of me; I did not need a Program. One night, the man who is my sponsor today called me and asked, "are you going to the Meeting tonight?" "No," I replied, "I thought I would go to a movie." There was a long pause. "Well," he said, "next time you feel like a drink, go to a movie." Then he hung up.

I went to the Meeting.

Pride can induce a drought, especially spiritual pride, the worst form of self-will. I was proud of my sobriety. There were no more issues to be solved. I was dispensing advice to anyone and everyone, whether they wanted it or not. I was active in service work. I had sponsees and loved to fix them. I would get into a snit if they did not pay me the proper amount of respect. I was losing track of everything that had gotten me that far. More and more, I was off the spiritual beam. I found my old friends, anger and fear. I remember one business meeting when I was off the beam. It was a board meeting for a treatment centre. I objected to the colour of the new carpet or something equally trivial. I still shudder at the recollection. Exploding in anger, I pounded the table and began shouting at him, displaying an ungentlemanly temper that was astounding. The other board members were stunned. Spiritual pride and independence from God, sheesh. That period did not end until after many Step Ten amends forced me to conclude that once again, my life was unmanageable.

I started the Steps again.

For some, AA becomes irritating. I have had many sponsees who, after attending hundreds of Meetings and hearing thousands of stories, concluded that they had nothing more to learn. The Meetings were a grind, hearing How It Works one more time was boring; they were irritated at the whiny yoga instructor's share and didn't care who had another bad day. They started arriving late and leaving early. Soon they were skipping Meetings. Sometimes I never saw them again.

Finally, we have the cranky Long-Timer. Cranky Long-Timers end up in the same place, but the roads they take may vary. One of my periods began when I walked into a Meeting feeling down and spiritually disconnected, but thinking that I had to have my game face on for the Meeting. After all, I had decades of sobriety; I had to appear happy, joyous and free; I was the old man at the Meeting; I could not show weakness; I had to attract. One game-faced Meeting led to another; it was tiring to maintain. I got crankier and crankier. Instead of happy, joyous, and free, I was becoming prickly, difficult, and gridlocked. Looking good made me feel bad. It made me cranky. I had to start sharing with my sponsor, and that broke the logjam. Sharing with him prepared me to share at Meetings. First sharing the problem, then sharing the solution.

Whatever the cause, if it goes unidentified or untreated, spiritual droughters leave the Rooms. They lose their Program.

Some drink and they are in real trouble, for they have tried the Program, and it failed them. They might feel doomed, refusing to go back to the Program they believe failed them.

Those who don't drink also have a steep path back to the Rooms. Life gets worse and worse. Some end it all. Rather than drink or come back, they commit suicide.

Those who do come back are to be admired. Like my new friend, they have swallowed hard and admitted they need help. Not driven by the lash of alcohol, which can excuse so many sins, they walk into the Rooms, sober and unhappy, and admit that they need help. That is courage.

That is why I start these GEMS with notes about Long-Term Sobriety. It is an area of our Program that we often ignore. We thank the Old-Timers for coming to Meetings and Round-Ups. But we don't pay attention to the issues around Old-Timers. What are we doing to encourage Old-Timers?

Several chapters of GEMS follow the section about Old-Timers: Serenity and Growth, the Steps, Self-Will and Ego, Inventories (the core of my Program) and then some fun with words; acronyms and word play.

You may read the whole book, or you may read one GEM at a time.

You may scan the chapter headings, and if one catches your eye, you might read some GEMS in that chapter. Still others, looking for something more specific, may scan the 'tags' and if a word catches their attention, dive into the GEMS that are connected with that tag.

However you approach or re-approach these GEMS, I hope and pray that some blessing is passed on to you, dear reader. For it is in giving it away that we get it more fully.

Longer-Term AA

Introduction

Some of us have been sober AA's for more than half our lives. Many of us have more years of sobriety than either Bill W. or Dr. Bob, our beloved founders. At AA World Conferences, the definition of Old-Timer is now 50 years of sobriety.

There is a lot of Long-Term Sobriety.

But Long-Timers are not the same as Old-Timers.

Long-Timers have many years. Old-Timers have much wisdom. Some Long-Timers have stalled. They have stalled in different ways. Some have repeated one year's sobriety five times. Others have repeated ten years' sobriety two or three times. Some are tired of Meetings. Some have lost touch with AA friends. Others are exhausted from having to show up at Meetings with a 'happy game face' even though they are anything but happy. So, they stop going to Meetings; they drift away from the Program. Many who are still involved have become grumpy and unattractive.

Old-Timers are blessed. They continued to grow, either by choice or necessity.

Some have read Bill's famous Grapevine article on Emotional Sobriety[1] and chosen to take his lessons to heart; establishing and continuing habits of spiritual maintenance that reflect their years of seniority. With this spiritual maintenance, they continue to spiritually grow and mature. To paraphrase the Good Book, "when they were newly sober, they ate and spoke

---

[1] The chapter entitled "Love" in As Bill Sees It, Grapevine.

as children, but they have put away childish things and now eat and speak of things of greater substance."

Others have had no choice. Significant life setbacks have caused enough pain, and they have had to grow spiritually or die, thereby blessed with a renewed Gift of Desperation.

Those who can claim to be Old-Timers are coming to the Rooms and sponsoring, and working the Steps in all their affairs. This is good. But many have also experienced the pains of spiritual pride; spiritual, the most dangerous pride of all.

This chapter is dedicated to Old-Timers; Long-timers who can become Old-Timers; and Old-Timers who have come to know the awful truth about spiritual pride.

Right and Wrong Questions

Tagged: #love, #program, #thinking, #unconditional, #wives

Often, I ask the wrong questions, which guarantees the wrong answers.

I ask wrong questions like: *Why can't I treat everyone with unconditional love? Why do I find it so hard to apply these principles in all my affairs? Why did God design me this way; could He not have created me to always think of the other guy first?*

I got nowhere. I was asking for the how and why of spiritual life. I was demanding explanations.

I need questions that reorient and adjust my attitudes and perceptions. I have to stop asking for explanations and start asking questions that stimulate changes in my attitudes and perceptions.

Questions like: *Am I thinking first about the other fellow? Am I consciously aware of the fact that God loves even my worst enemy? Am I applying these principles in all my affairs? Am I consciously aware of God right now? What actions am I taking to be mindful of God?*

Asking these questions on the fly during the day is good, but a great start to the day is better. The "on awakening" checklists, on pages 86 and 87 of the Big Book stimulate right actions. The checklists that I have developed and published on the4thdimension.ca based on these simple directions start things off with the right questions. Look under the Worksheets tab on the Home Page for the Daily Checklists.

The morning and evening checklists take a minute to complete. The questions do not point my mind to a demand for explanations. They point my mind to right actions, attitudes and perceptions.

It is so simple. But it requires discipline.

Good habits — Bad habits
Tagged: #good and evil, #habits, #spiritual growth

I worry about why bad habits seem more natural and more comfortable than good habits.

It is true, bad habits develop quickly and are difficult to dislodge; conversely, keeping good habits requires persistence; they are easily lost.

Example — morning meditations. Hard to habituate and easy to stop. How many times do I have to learn the lessons of the value of a morning meditation and period of prayer? I get on the beam and practice this habit for a time. I become aware that the days that start with a good morning meditation seem to go better. Then one morning, I decide that ten minutes more sleep would be better than a morning meditation. Soon my morning prayer and meditation habits are gone.

The same pattern, of hard to start and easy to lose, is found with my evening review of the day. I get tired one night and go to bed without doing my daily review; then the habit is gone.[2]

Why are good habits hard to acquire and easy to lose; and bad habits easy to get and hard to lose? Maybe there is an evil force in nature. This force drives out good habits and embeds bad habits. A variation of "the devil made me do it." Sometimes I think it is the way that we are wired. God seems to have wired us with a bias to the wrong way of doing things. Is God testing us with temptations? Who knows? But I ponder these problems.

---

[2] For copies of the checklists that I use in the morning and evening, go to the4thdimension.ca and look under Worksheets.

Then I stop and realize that the reasons good habits are easy to lose and bad habits are easy to get are not essential to solving the problem. The problem is solved with actions, not thoughts. The actions are the Steps of our Program, the principles we practice in our lives. Actions like: pray and meditate, do an inventory, pause and turn to God when disturbed or deciding, help someone else, help someone in the Program. Take the required actions. "Just do it." Who cares about why the bad seems stronger than the good? Accept that I seem to find it hard to get good habits and easy to get bad habits; or easy to lose good habits and hard to drop bad habits. What good is the explanation?

Actions are the key, not theories. What is needed is persistence and hard work. The actions embedded in the Steps are guides for the persistence and hard work that I need.

Checking out your Serenity

Tagged: #acceptance, #serenity

I heard a great line at a Meeting: "If you are in the express line at the grocery store and the person in front of you has more than the permitted number of items in their basket and you say nothing, you have acceptance. If you don't even count the number of items in their basket, you have serenity."

This is a great way to measure serenity, but it lacks sophistication and nuance. I wanted to expand upon this to create a powerful self-evaluation tool. I wanted to find a way to measure acceptance and serenity in a more detailed manner. After all, if it is important you should measure it, and if you want to manage it, you have to measure it. We need a proper scoring mechanism for acceptance and serenity, the two foundations for a good AA life.

If anyone in front of you has more than the permitted number of items (and you are guaranteed to have one) and you make a comment to your neighbour in line, stare hard, or snort with derision, Acceptance—0, Serenity—0.

If you count the items in the basket of someone in front of you and roll your eyes, but say nothing and make no noises, Acceptance—3, Serenity—0.

If you count the items and exercising iron discipline, you do nothing and make no noises, Acceptance—5, Serenity—3.

If you don't count the number of items of anyone in front of you, Acceptance—5, Serenity—5.

It is in the little situations that mean nothing, like those private moments in the check-out line, thinking about those in front who are wronging us, that we discover how we are doing.

We should aim for five by five scores. Especially in the little things.

Separating the men from the boys

Tagged: #emotional sobriety, #spiritual growth, #step 12, #steps

Long-timers become Old-Timers because they mature; not because they grow old.

Bill W., in a letter to his spiritual sponsor, Father Ed Dowling, discussed Steps Six and Seven of our Program. He wrote, "these steps separate the 'men from the boys' all right. But if a 'man' is to be defined as one who is perfectly and continuously willing (to have defects removed), then the number of them must be quite small. I am inclined to define the 'man' as the one who has arrived at the point where he can try to be willing in all respects without being whiplashed into it by dire necessity."

This thought lends an interesting dimension to the idea of Steps Six and Seven being the point of "separation of the men from the boys."

When I first came to the Rooms of AA, I had the Gift of Desperation that whiplashed me into the Program.

Later, I turned to the Steps again, but under the compulsion of dire necessity. I was not drinking, but I was still power driving and self-centred. Life's problems were driving me to conclude that I had to change, so I turned to the Steps, but only because I was whiplashed into it.

As the years passed and I began to experience the positive effects of character development, I progressed to the point where every once in a while I would take the Steps in regards to a defect of character without the lash of the whip, or the Gift of Desperation. Every once in a while, I would do something to improve my character without a crisis. Every once in a while, I would invest some time in character building when things were running all right. I started to realize the value of character building, over and above crisis management.

With these small character improvements, I could claim some modicum of manhood. By Bill's definition, I was maturing.

Thankfully, the Gift of Desperation is still available. There are still defects which I identify and resolve, driven by the lash of the whip, and the Gift of Desperation. But with my annual inventory processes, quarterly reviews, and daily prayer and meditation habits, I can identify character defects, give them names, and, with God, work on them before the whipping starts; or at least before a crisis erupts.

But this requires daily, quarterly, and annual disciplines of inventory. Like any good business, periodic inventories are required. Confessional conversations about the results of the inventory to identify the exact nature of the problem are also necessary; then, of course, as night follows day, so is working with God to remove them.

I am not claiming that I am separated from the boys, but at least once in a while, I peer over the fence into manhood.

Are you still waiting for the lash of the whip to take a next spiritual step? Then grow up. You can stop the pain.

Static Build-Up in My Head

Tagged: #anger, #growing up, #spiritual growth, #nowhere

For me, anger was a problem. Rages frequently blew up in my life. I never seemed to see them coming. My temper would explode without warning and, to all appearances, randomly.

It seemed like a bolt of lightning striking without warning. This metaphor bears consideration. Though lightning strikes may appear to be arbitrary, they develop in a predictable manner and the strikes are far from random. Rules of nature govern them.

It all begins long before the actual strike, with the interaction of charged particles in a cloud. Massive energy is built up in a thunderhead with little electrons swirling, mixing, and bumping against each other, creating an electric charge. The charge builds and builds until, suddenly, it bursts out in a dramatic lightning strike.

The location of the strike appears to be random, but it follows rules. Clouds move. The charge buildup might have been over a wheat field, but the discharge might happen when the cloud is over a village. When the wind blew the cloud over the village, the lightning struck the nearest (highest) target that it could find.

So this apparently violent and random event has a development cycle that we can understand, and strike location rules that can be predicted.

My temper tantrums are the same. They appear to be random and without warning, but there are development cycles that can be understood and patterns and rules that are followed.

Anger builds up in my forehead. Like little electrons in a thunderhead cloud, minor irritations swirl and mix, bumping against each other, creating an emotional charge. Then when the emotional charge has built up enough, suddenly without warning, it bursts out.

Like a thunderhead cloud building a charge over a wheat field and discharging it over a village, the charge in my forehead might build up at work, then the strike hits when I arrive at home. No matter where the charge builds up, when it strikes, it looks for the most convenient target at that moment.

The rage seems to appear from nowhere. But when I do a personal inventory, the buildup of the emotional charge at the office is evident. I can discern the exact cause of the build-up. I can see that the target was just the highest and most convenient target at the time of the strike.

I cannot stop lightning strikes from thunderheads. Mother Nature will go on, but with inventories and reliance upon God, I can understand and stop my rages.

Maintaining a conscious contact with my Higher Power can prevent the phenomenon. The little irritations don't swirl and mix and bump against each other, creating an emotional charge. Even if a small charge builds up, conscious contact with my Higher Power neutralizes the charge within my forehead. The rages never occur.

Wow. What a blessing the Steps are in my life.

Atheist spirituality

Tagged: #agnostics, #judging in the program, #spiritual awakening, #spiritual growth, #step 10

Years of sobriety are not determinative of an AA's quality of sobriety and spiritual maintenance. I learned that from many who have been in the Rooms for less time than I.

There is a woman who attends my Home Group. She has fewer years than I, but often has a better message.

This is her story. As an atheist, she came to the AA Program and over time came to see that a spiritual dimension could work in her life. Her words are a great comfort to the many newcomers who might otherwise be put off by me and my God messages, my references to the need for spiritual growth and the presence of God in my life.

Now don't get me wrong; I hope that some in the room want to hear my message, which tends to focus more on awareness of a Higher Power, God. But her message may be more important to the raw recruit, and I can take a lesson from her.

Bill W. announced early on, after about three or four years, that the Akron crowd was doing much better than the New York crowd, because the Akronites emphasized the spiritual angle. He suggested that it was time for the New York AA's to emphasize spirituality more. Fifteen years later, he wrote that too many newcomers were turned off by the preacher tone in many of the Rooms. He was struggling to find the right balance in the Rooms.

It seems to me that my friend in my Home Group has hit the sweet spot. She talks about the spiritual angle, but as an atheist, her comments are surprising and gentle. She talks about her atheism combined with the simple actions of the Steps and the Fellowship. By emphasizing the actions over beliefs, she conveys the truth of the message without baggage; baggage that may be too heavy for some to carry.

She focuses on the idea that she is not God, and how that simple door allowed her to pass through to new ideas.

I am not an atheist, but I can tailor my message to better fit the virgin ear of the newcomer. Start simple, share that I learned that I am not God by doing the Steps outlined in our basic text. Things can go from there.

Be gentle and trust in the process.

When is God in your life?

Tagged: #alarms, #*awareness*, #*God as I understood Him*, #*spiritual growth*, #*meditation*, #*step 11*

Bill W points out that either God is everything, or He is nothing.

If He is everything, then I should be thinking about Him all through the day. After all, He is in charge of the whole universe. If I believe He is guiding me, I should be consciously aware of Him. And not just once in a while, but all the time. He is a force to be reckoned with; I should, in theory, be occupied with nothing else.

But I cannot seem to meet that standard. Never mind maintaining continuous contact with God; I can't seem to manage periodic contact with God.

In my nightly inventory, I review the day and ask myself, "During the day, was I consciously aware of God?" I often have to answer, "Not really" or "Not very often."

I might start well in the morning. Immediately after my morning meditation, I am thinking about Him and I am aware of His presence. By lunchtime, I have little conscious awareness of God. In the afternoon, I have forgotten Him completely.

The creator of the universe, the Being that has all power – I have forgotten Him. What is with that?

And this forgetfulness of God is curious; there is no excuse. I know I can focus on things for long stretches. With other subjects, I can concentrate. For example, I have dwelt on business or legal problems for long periods of time. I can focus on important clients and their needs for days. I can obsess for hours about slights, wrongs, and insults that I perceive have been aimed at me. I am a guy, so I can think about sex throughout the day.

I know from experience that I can focus on things for a long time, so why can't I think about God with that same tenacity? Why can't I focus on God the way I focus on sex, clients, legal problems, and resentments?

I needed to learn to habituate thinking about God. I read a book about habits, and it suggested that I create triggers to initiate a good habit. This seemed like a good idea.

I decided to use technology as a trigger. I set up alarms on my phone. Silent, and labelled with short reminders to turn my mind to God. I have five alarms set: mid-morning, just before lunch; mid-afternoon; later afternoon; and two during the evening. Each label is a different four- or five-word reminder of some aspect of God. Labels like:

- God is in this;

- God is here and now;

- God loves you;

- God is aware of you; and,

- Be mindful of God.

The alarm goes off; the label comes up; I am reminded to be consciously aware of God.

Five times a day, I am reminded to turn my mind to God. Sometimes I stop to think about the label, but even if I don't, I am briefly made consciously aware of God; enough to turn towards Him.

On this foundation of habit, I am building a higher frequency of conscious awareness of God throughout the day.

Michaelangelo or Mickey Mouse

Tagged: #spiritual growth, #removing defects, #step 6, #step 7

I have always had a spiritual thirst.

Before I came into the Program, I had a series of born-again religious experiences. I accepted Jesus as my saviour, and all my sins were forgiven in the twinkling of an eye. I was promised that if I gave my life to Jesus, I would be magically transformed.

When I think of these experiences, I am reminded of Mickey Mouse in the classic Disney cartoon, *Fantasia*. Dressed in a wizard's robe, Mickey waved his magic wand, and everything he touched was transformed; objects exploded with colour, stars were sprinkled in the skies. That is what I was promised. A magic wand would touch me and explode with spiritual colour.

When I came to AA, I found a new path. No Mickey Mouse here, no magic wands either; I had to ask God to remove defects of character.

The new path was like Michelangelo, who was asked, "How did you create the great statue of David?"he is reported to have said, "Every block of stone has a statue inside it and it is the task of the sculptor to discover it." David had been underneath all along.

Michelangelo removed marble to reveal David. God is removing defects to reveal Andy.

But removing marble is messy work — big hammers and chisels for the larger pieces, transitioning to noisy smaller chisels for the smaller bits, and finally finishing with dusty sanding and grinding. That is the Program way, the Michelangelo way. It is dirty, noisy and messy. It is hard work.

Mickey Mouse touched something with his wand, and it was transformed. Michelangelo worked hard to chisel and sand away the marble, and a new shape emerged.

Interestingly, the Mickey Mouse colours quickly faded, but the reshaped marble was permanently revealed.

Which would I have, a Micky Mouse and his wand, or God and His character chisels? I think God is the better bet.

Putting boundaries on recovery

Tagged: #emotional sobriety, #spiritual growth, #spiritual awakening, #step 2

Last week, a speaker at the Haddon Road group in Calgary said that she had put boundaries on her Program. I recognized that I had done the same thing.

When I first came into AA, I limited the Program to my drinking. It worked. The desire to drink was lifted from me. But I stopped there. I felt like I had reached a boundary.

Later, I saw that my Program did not have to be limited to my drinking. Here is the story.

First, I discovered recurring defects of character. With regular Step Ten inventories, I saw patterns, the same mistakes over and over. Defects of character were repeated again and again. It seemed that I had no control over them. Like the drinker who finds himself with a drink in his hand and wonders how it got there, I repeated these character defects thoughtlessly and carelessly.

Of course, after inventorying the wrong, I have to admit it. In the first inventory, when I saw the wrong, I was pointed to the word 'admit' in Step Five. I would admit the wrong to another human being. Sometimes just saying, "I am sorry." But when I repeated the wrongs, and these patterns were revealed in my regular inventories, I was pointed to the word 'admit' in Step One. I was forced to admit that I was powerless. My powerlessness was evidenced by the thoughtless and repetitive nature of the mistakes. These behaviours were making my life unmanageable.

Starting at Step One with these admissions, the next indicated Step was coming to believe that the problem was between my ears, not my circumstances. My thinking was not clean; it was not sane. Also, I had to come to believe that a Power greater than myself could restore me to clean thinking.

Then, with this Step One and Two start, I could begin to practice the Steps in my life, on these wrongs identified in inventories.

With the application of the Steps to other problems, I extended my Program's boundaries. I extended the Program beyond drinking and into more of my affairs.

Serenity and growth

Introduction

In the Rooms of AA, we talk about serenity and spiritual growth. We desire serenity and want to grow spiritually.

But for years, I defaulted to my factory settings, which were not aimed at serenity or spiritual growth. My factory settings were aimed at feeling good and inflating my Ego. I had to change my settings away from my Ego to my character, and from feeling good to accepting life. This process of resetting myself to desire character and increased self-esteem required attention and effort.

Changing my settings was not something that I could do myself. It required power. My dilemma was the lack of power. Not being able to do it myself, the power had to come from an outside source. I needed a Power other than myself and it had to be greater than mine; I had to take the advice of that Power, to acknowledge that when it came to my mental settings, it was the higher authority.

I had to admit that I needed a Power greater than myself, and I had to believe that Power could, if asked, restore me to proper thinking, a change of my mental settings.

Mouthing platitudes and repeated wishing will not do the trick.

Serenity and growth required desire and effort. They require a will to believe.

These GEMS are notes on these points.

I hope you enjoy them.

Emotional Sobriety

Tagged: #emotional sobriety, #spiritual awakening, #spiritual growth, #step 10, #inventory, #subsequent awakenings

Recently, I attended a Meeting named Emotional Sobriety. The theme of the Meeting was Emotional Sobriety as Bill W. described it in the 12 x 12, and in a famous Grapevine article, reprinted in *The Best of Bill*.[3]

He referred to Emotional Sobriety as the next level of growth in AA, both individually and corporately. Bill W. described his own experiences in both finding and growing Emotional Sobriety.

Since then, I have discovered several Meetings with similar themes. Two common names for these Meetings are the Second Awakening and Awakenings. These names seem to me to be appropriate. Emotional Sobriety, in my experience, comes with the second, third, and subsequent spiritual awakenings.

As I see it, in Step 12, we are promised a first spiritual awakening as the result of these Steps. But my experience confirms that after this first spiritual awakening, we can have a second, third, fourth, and more spiritual awakenings.

The first spiritual awakening was sufficient to stop drinking; I managed to stop and stay stopped. A survey of the Steps, persistent attendance at Meetings, and service work were enough to keep me sober. This time of mere sobriety was followed by a long plateau of no or little growth. During this period, even though I had experienced one small spiritual awakening, my personality and behaviours reflected my untreated alcoholism and lack of spiritual growth. All I had done was to plug the jug. I was still sick and off my medication,

---

[3] The chapter entitled "Love" in the Best of Bill, published by Grapevine Publishing.

booze. My anger and temper manifested frequently, both at work and home. I continued my self-centred and prideful attitudes and perceptions, causing discomfort to those around me.

Admittedly I wasn't drinking. But, to show how bad things got — one day, the office manager in our law firm approached me and explained that it was becoming impossible for her to find legal assistants to work with me. I was too angry and difficult and the word had spread. And this was after some years off the booze.

Who cares, I thought to myself; I was succeeding. I was a young lawyer, and my billings were high. The partners were happy, and I understood which side of the bread the butter was on. Clients enjoyed working with me, but junior lawyers and secretaries whom I worked with, not so much.

Sober up a drunken horse thief, all you have is a sober horse thief. While drinking, I was a drunken angry man. After I stopped drinking, I was a sober, angry man. I was a power driver whose success was self-derived.

The next spiritual awakenings allowed me to grow to higher levels of spiritual thought and feeling, what I now think of as Emotional Sobriety.

Any Emotional Sobriety that I gained came through these subsequent spiritual awakenings. These awakenings materialized as a result of working the Steps. The period where I attended Meetings without applying the Steps was a difficult time, but over many years of Meetings, and seeing others live increasingly serene and calm lives, I began to perceive the results of working the Steps. I noticed, in the Big Book, how often the words persistence and hard work were used when talking about the Steps. I began applying perseverance and hard work to the Steps and myself. I started to live the last half of Step 12, "practising these principles in all our affairs."

I worked the Steps and baked them into my life, and it paid off. Persistent application of the Steps to problems in my life, became my Program of spiritual maintenance. Slowly but surely over the decades, my level of spiritual growth and Emotional Sobriety has increased.

I had successive spiritual awakenings as a result of those Steps.

As the Big Book states on page 14, "Belief in the power of God, plus enough willingness, honesty and humility to establish and maintain the new order of things, were the essential requirements. Simple, but not easy; a price had to be paid. It meant the destruction of self-centeredness."

And this destruction requires the persistent application of the Steps. At least that is my story.

Hallmark of Fear

Tagged: #shame, #dependence, #self centred, #abandon, #businessman on the beach, #spiritual awakening, #growth, #fear, #denial

"One of the hallmarks of a life run on self-will is fear."[4]

When my life is running on self-will, I am relying on myself, and I am frequently in a state of fear.

When we do not depend on God and cannot depend on anyone else, we are absolutely alone. Unconsciously we realize this, and two things result: we more easily become afraid, and the fear is more deep-seated than normal.

For example, we are not just afraid of failure; we are fearful of the possibility of failure. Relying on our own resources and dependent on our frail selves, we are scared because we know how weak we are, and failure seems likely. Fear comes more easily.

And the severity of the fear is more profound because failure becomes existential, life-threatening. When something goes wrong or works out differently from what I expect, then it is a threat to my being. I have willed something to be so, and it is not working out that way. It is my judgment and will-power that is being denied; success and failure are judgments on my will and my power. Because I am entirely dependent upon myself, it all rests upon me, and my will and my power are all that is holding this part of the universe together. This anxiety and fear threaten my personality, my core. The failure is a failure of my very being.

I remember meeting with some clients and a takeover target. The clients had never been involved in a takeover. I was sure

---

[4] Quoted from a Joe and Charlie tape.

that they were looking to me for leadership on the project. After all, I had done it once before. Before the meeting, I mapped out the conversation that I expected on a piece of paper. Full of confidence and Ego, I walked into the board room. I did not pause, pray, and listen for my Higher Power. I had a lot of years of sobriety but forgot to include God in my thinking, maybe I assumed He knew nothing about corporate takeovers. I was on my own.

We sat down and I started the conversation.

A world heavyweight boxer said once "Everyone has a plan on how to fight me, but that goes out the window with the first punch in the head." Well, in that meeting, I experienced a verbal punch in the head. The takeover target had hired an experienced and well-known lawyer. The takeover target was not amused by the prospect and their lawyer made that clear. In front of my clients, the more experienced lawyer accused me of incompetence and being an amateur. I was on my own, and knowing how little experience I had, I was paralyzed in fear. The fear went right to my core. I imagined the loss of clients, being dismissed from the firm and losing my law licence. And that was in the first three seconds. The fear was instantaneous and existential. I was sick to my stomach.

So I have learned, if a situation causes that type of fear, there is a good chance that I am depending upon myself.

Pre-flight checklist

Tagged: #checklist, #discipline, #spiritual growth, #habits, #spiritual awakening, #step 10

Years ago, I was working with a fellow AA. He was having issues.

He was a pilot. Now I don't know a lot about flying, but I do know that pilots use checklists. So I asked him, "As a pilot, would you ever think of landing or taking off without using your takeoff and landing checklist?"

He said, "Of course not."

I then asked him why he thought he could take off in the morning for the day and land in the evening, going to bed without going through his checklist. We then went to look for any checklists that Bill W. had designed. Sure enough, in the Big Book, we find the daily checklists. On pages 86-87, Bill suggests questions that are the checklists for taking off in the morning and landing in the evening.

My friend thought this was a brilliant idea. So did I. I went home and built two checklists based on the page 86-87 questions.

I use my checklists two times each day, morning and evening — takeoff and landing.

It does not take long; the propositions found on page 86 and 87 are short and powerful.

The morning checklist sets up the day. The propositions make me mindful of God.

The evening checklist eases my mind to allow me a good sleep. The propositions make me mindful of God in my life.

I have found my checklists to be a useful tool, one that has helped me grow in the sunlight of the spirit.[5]

---

[5] My checklists can be found on my website, the4thdimension.ca, under Worksheets. Feel free to use them and adjust them to fit your situation.

Host to God or Slave to My Ego, Part 1

Tagged: #God as I understood Him, #spiritual awakening, #step 3

Host to God or Slave to my Ego? I heard this AA saying at a Meeting recently. This AA aphorism captures a vital nuance of spiritual life.

The initial choice offered is between Hosting and Slavery.

Hosting is hard; it takes time and effort. Hosting a dinner party means sending invitations, setting the table and laying out the food, etc. Hosting God also takes effort — prayer, meditation, inventories, etc.

On the other hand, Slavery is easy; I surrender and give up, and without any further action, I am a Slave, ready to follow orders. It is a one and done solution. One simple decision, and I am a Slave. Becoming a Slave to my Ego is effortless. Once my Ego switches on and occupies centre stage, I just let my Ego take over; it is the new Master, and I am a Slave. With one decision, my Ego takes over. I don't have to think about it; it just takes over.

The choice is between a lot of work and effort on the one hand; and an easy, one and done decision on the other. The work and effort to Host is the correct choice; it appears harder than the second. But trust me, as you will see in the next GEM, it is easier.

Host to God or Slave to My Ego, Part 2

Tagged: #dependence, #self centred, #ego, #self will, #emotional sobriety, #conscious awareness, #self-centered, #growing up, #habits, #dependency on the opinion of others, #tools of the program, #awareness

As we saw in the last GEM, it is more work and effort to be a Host than to become a Slave.

But once that decision is made, it takes more effort to be a Slave than to become a Host

Hosting God is easy. God, as I have understood Him, is not a hard Guest to entertain. As a Guest, He offers care and protection, not command and control. In Step Three, we turn our will and our lives over to the care of God; we seek His care and protection. The proposed relationship is gentle; care and protection are the watchwords.

The proof of the pudding, as they say, is in the eating. When I Host God, things seem to work out better. When I take the time and effort to align my thoughts with God by becoming consciously aware of him, I tend to see things more clearly and comprehensively; and that in turn leads me to make correct decisions more often. Hosting God is easy work.

But being a Slave to my Ego is hard work. In my experience, immediately upon becoming a Slave, the real work, effort, and pain begin. There are judgments to be made, tempers to flare, energy to expend chasing things around. It is hard work. There is a lot to think about. Since I am in control, I have to arrange a lot of pieces on the board. Controlling them is tough. The players often have minds of their own. If that were not enough, there are lies to be told and truths to be managed. Then there are consequences to face and amends to be made; the work is never-ending.

Today, I will make an effort to Host God. Today I will try to remember that it is harder to Host, but God is a comfortable Guest. It is easier to become a Slave, but my Ego is a hard Master.

Rule of Three Ups

Tagged: #growing up, #program, #spiritual awakening, #steps

At a recent Meeting, I heard an aphorism that is true for alcoholics of our type; the Rule of Three Ups.

We have three options when we are drinking:

1. We can die and be covered **up**,

2. We can become insane and be locked **up**, or

3. We can come to AA and sober **up**.

There is the second Rule of Three Ups that applies after we come into the Program.

1. We can freeze **up**,

2. We can slip **up**, or

3. We can grow **up**.

At first, coming to the Meetings kept me sober. But I did not get a sponsor. I was not reading the Big Book or working the Steps. I froze up. I had a great Fellowship, lots of AA friends and community and service work, but a terrible Program. Spiritually I was frozen.

I had this frozen Program for a long time, and I had five years in the Rooms, but I had repeated the first year five times, staying sober but acting like the unmedicated alcoholic I had become. I suffered through this, and since then, I have seen many others go through the same phase.

Fortunately, I didn't slip up, like so many others. But if you are frozen in your Program, then the time may come when Meetings and Fellowship get old, and the connection with AA slips away; then you are heading for a slip-up. Even if you don't slip up, a freeze-up period is uncomfortable, both for you and people around you. You can survive and not drink, but it is not fun.

Eventually, I started to grow up. I started working the Steps. I started in my sixth year of sobriety; I took one year and did a Step per month. The next year, I began a habit of an annual inventory and confessional conversation with my spiritual advisor. I start this process each year on my AA birthday. I also started some new daily habits. I habituated my daily meditation and prayer habits and diarized regular interactions with my sponsor to check in and monitor my progress. I started working on conscious awareness of God during the day. I was blessed with sponsees and began working with them to study the Steps.

With these habits, I thawed my "freeze up," avoided a "slip up," and began to "grow up."

Find Serenity — Pray for the Son of a Bitch

Tagged: *#amends, #anger, #measurement of results, #prayer, #spiritual awakening, #stories*

After coming to AA, I had to acknowledge the reality of my anger. Up until that point, you might have said that I was in denial. It did not seem like denial. I did not see it and consciously reject it. Instead, I just didn't see it, and if I did see it, I did not understand it.

But regardless, it was there. I was an angry young man. Newly sober, starting my career, I became embroiled in a personality clash at work. I became crazy angry. Without the medicative effect of booze, I could not find any relief.

I talked to my sponsor. He told me "I have only been that angry with one person in sobriety, and the solution hurt so much I never got that angry again… the solution was painful and difficult… I had to pray for the son of a bitch; I had to talk honestly to God about him."

So I prayed about him. I did not pray *for* him, just *about* him. I talked with God about him every morning, as my sponsor had instructed me. I started the first morning on my knees. I decided to be honest. God knows everything, I thought, so He already knew what was in my heart. Asking for a blessing for this character was BS and God knew it. Declaring my love for him was even worse. I pointed out to God that He should not take my prayers for the asshole as approval of him or his behaviour. I recall telling God, "You are supposed to be perfect in all that you do, but when you created this guy, you made a mistake."

After one week of daily prayers, my opinion was unchanged, but my conversation with God changed, I found myself saying, "God… my opinion of him is unchanged, but if it is necessary that something good happen to him for the proper unfolding of your universe… so be it."

Over the following days, the language of my conversations with God changed to a grudging, "Okay, he is your creation, and though I still think you screwed up in creating him, please bless him, and if possible, let something good happen to him today."

It worked; the relationship changed. The anger magically dissipated and was replaced with a general sense of impartial goodwill.[6] The relationship had been amended, made right.

This small experience shows me the path to serenity. To be willing to seek and take advice from a spiritual advisor, then taking indicated actions whether I believed they would work or not.

---

[6] This is the definition of love that was developed by Emmet Fox.

Into Actions

Tagged: #checklist, #morning checklist, #step 11, #morning meditation

Take the actions — I can act my way into a new way of thinking.

The chapter in The Big Book is "Into Action," not "Into Prayer" or "Into Thought." Actions are the key. Bring the body, and the heart and mind will follow.

Here is an example from my life. For years, I have habituated a morning and evening routine; the routine includes checklists. On my iPad there are boxes to tick off for each completed item. The checklists are derived from the questions posed on pages 86-87 of the Big Book. The worksheets can be found on my website. Feel free to download them, at the4thdimension.ca.

But here is the problem: Daily repetition can drain meaning. Many nights and mornings, these checklists seem formulaic. Asking myself the same questions every day and ticking off the boxes every day is not a very exciting activity. Frankly, many days, I don't even think about the questions, never mind form a deep awareness of them. So, does merely doing them make a difference, or do I have to think deeply about the questions?

At times, I have allowed the practice to lapse — I begin to think, "I can go to sleep early tonight, I don't need to do my checklist." I have had stretches of days and weeks of doing these checklists every day, and periods of not doing these checklists.

Some years ago, I conducted a controlled experiment. I did the checklists faithfully for several weeks and tracked the days and informally scored each day on a sentiment and satisfaction scale of 1-10. I did not spend more time on the checklists; I treated them like the everyday occurrence they were, surfing through them quickly. Then I stopped the checklist habit for a time and likewise scored the days.

Sure enough, when I am habitually doing my simple checklists, life goes better. I score higher on my satisfaction and sentiment scores — I feel better. Coincidentally I make more money (better decisions), have fewer arguments (reductions in both scope and frequency), find more parking spots (they just seem to appear as I wait), and I meet fewer idiot drivers on the roadways (I let them get in front of me and they drive away).

So, I don't need to feel meaning or depth when asking the questions in my checklists. I can surf through them quickly. But I do need to do them. I need to complete the actions.

Much like the sponsee who whined that he could not pray on his knees because "he did not believe in God."

The sponsor replied, "You don't have to believe in anything; you just have to do it. Get down on your knees and say you need help. That's all. Just do it."

Weeks later the sponsee admitted that it "seemed to be making a difference."

We have the most ruthlessly pragmatic theology in the world. If it works, we do it, and if not, we stop.

My God is a very practical God.

If You Spot It, You Got It

Tagged: #inventory, #step 10

A good friend, from San Diego, where there is excellent AA, reminded me of a superb AA slogan: "You Spot It, You Got It."

Sometimes, I think this should be on a poster in the Rooms, right beside "Think Think Think."

We were having a coffee together. He shared that several things were irritating him about someone we both knew.

I observed that often, when I criticized someone for an act, word or deed; later, I would see that I was guilty of the same action, word, or deed.

If a sponsee annoyed me by holding on to some belief that was not working, sure enough, I was doing the same thing. If someone cut me off in traffic, a flash of irritation zipped through me, and a few minutes later, I would cut somebody else off. If someone made a joke at my expense, the flash of anger was soon followed by my making a joke at someone else's expense. If I was irritated by a gossiper or name dropper, when I thought for a moment, I was doing or had done the same thing.

If I saw somebody doing something I did not like, I realized I was doing the same thing.

Over and over, this pattern repeated. Behaviours that I found irritating in others were behaviours of mine that I found offensive.

He laughed and said, "If you spot it, you got it."

Spiritual Naps

*Tagged: #spiritual growth, #persistence, #awareness of god,
#meditation*

I have had spiritual awakenings; then I lost them.

In Meetings, we often talk about turning our will and lives over
the to the care of God, then taking them back.

Sometimes I do that, but often it seems much more passive. I
did not seize my will back and wrest it from God's hands, I just
took a spiritual nap.

When I forget my morning and evening meditation and prayer
routines, I can feel my spiritual head begin to nod, the precursor
to a spiritual nap. I find my life does not run as smoothly. I
become irritated, restless, and discontented. That, I have
learned, is a signal to renew my meditation and prayer practices
to get back on the beam — to become consciously aware of my
Higher Power. I have to wake up from the nap.

So, taking my life back is one thing — but another is just having
a spiritual nap.

Push My Buttons — See What You Get

Tagged: #changes, #lack of power, #pushing buttons, #reacting to the world, #spiritual growth, #step 10

People are always pushing my buttons.

I walk around with buttons exposed to the world. Anyone can push them and get a reaction.

Each button feels different and provokes a different reaction. The back buttons feel good when pressed with hugs and slaps on the back. The chest buttons are mixed and sensitive; these can cause anger when you jab at my chest. The genital buttons are powerful; the reaction is immediate and dominating.

There are buttons that I expose to the world. There is one on my forehead, positioned so that I can stick it in your face. I dare you to push it; sometimes, I am eager for you to push it. Some buttons are hidden from sight and sometimes pushed by accident.

People who are close to me can push my buttons. They often know where they are located from past experience. Strangers are less familiar with my buttons, but they can press them nonetheless, they seem to stumble on them accidentally.

Some buttons are wired for a single reaction. Pushing the button opens a specific circuit of either pleasure; ease and politeness; or fear, anger, and irritation.

Other buttons are more confusing. They have multiple connections. They seem to be cross-wired to a mix of fear, anger, pride, together with pleasure, politeness, and ease. You will get different reactions from the same button. Like the "Can I help?" button. Press it, and you can randomly trigger either the "Bugger off, I got this" or the, "Yes please, could you help" response.

I used to think that I should disconnect all the wiring to my buttons with the Steps. Now I realize that with the Steps, I am not disconnecting the buttons, I am re-wiring the connections to the buttons. The same buttons that used to trigger anger and fear can be re-wired to be curious and polite. Buttons with confused wiring can be straightened out.

The best example is the "Why on earth did you do that?" button. It is right beside the "That was stupid" button, and sometimes people push both. My old wiring caused an adverse reaction with responses like: "Who are you to criticize me?" or "Who are you to question me?" After many explosive reactions, followed by inventories and amends, I learned that I could re-wire the circuits to respond differently. When the buttons were pushed, I could reply with: "That is interesting," or "That is one way of looking at things" or, best of all, "You might be right."

But re-wiring the buttons has to be done in advance of the button-pushing, and it requires hard work, practice, and the right tools. I have never been able to change my button reactions on the fly. I have to put in the hard work of Steps Six and Seven, with the continuous feedback of Step Ten, enforced with the discipline of Steps Eight and Nine to re-wire the buttons.

Lack of power was not my only dilemma; sometimes, bad wiring leads to badly directed power. Re-wiring my buttons with God's guidance helps. Re-wiring my buttons using the Steps gives me better reactions. Life is much more peaceful.

Morning Meditation

Tagged: #meditation, #spiritual growth, #daily habits, #dependence

I have a morning checklist, my 'take-off checklist' before launching myself for the day.[7]

All the questions in the morning checklist are good, but there is one that stands out. It is "Consider the day ahead." When I consider the day ahead, I think about meetings and telephone calls that are coming up through the day. I ask myself whether or not there is anything I need to be prepared for or be aware of. Do I need to consider the people involved and their feelings and interests? Do I need to brace myself for an awkward conversation? Do I need to honour and reward somebody? Should I thank someone for something?

If you looked up the word 'meditation' in a 1935 American dictionary, you would find that one of the meanings of 'meditation' is 'planning.' A businessman would meditate on his business plan. A general would meditate on his battle plan. Bill suggests that we meditate on our day ahead.

In discussing meditation, Bill does suggest a quiet contemplation that might look like Zen or Buddhist meditation. But he also suggests another, more active, dimension to meditation — planning for the day ahead. This latter dimension is the most practical and meaningful in my experience. It sets my day up well.

Every morning I look at my calendar. I make a short note about each meeting and phone call that I have booked. Later, when I look at the calendar, I see the note and I am reminded of my

---

[7] Check out the Worksheets on my website, the4thdimension.ca.

state of mind in my morning preparation, when I was fully mindful of God and His will for me.

When I pause and think about the day ahead, I am mentally and spiritually prepared to take on the day. If there are any surprises during the day, I am poised and ready for the unexpected.

You don't have to become a monk, chanting OM every morning. If you are having trouble with the whole Eastern meditation thing, try something from the Big Book. Try pausing and thinking about the day ahead. Try it for a couple of weeks. You will love it.

Being Where I Am

Tagged: #in the moment, #present

At a recent Meeting, a person sharing said, "I can choose to be where I am… or not."

I would change this to "I have to choose to be where I am… if I don't, I am not."

I have to choose to be aware and pay attention.

It might look like I am planning, but I am really daydreaming. I daydream, mistaking daydreaming for planning, deceived into thinking that it is useful. I occupy myself with fantasies of grandeur, material possessions, fame and fortune, sexual conquests, and even, I am ashamed to admit, delusions of spiritual magnificence. At those times, my lack of presence in the moment is astounding.

It may look like I am paying attention to you, but when I was first introduced to you, I didn't even hear your name because I was completely preoccupied with how I look, putting my best face forward. I am oblivious to you.

In Meetings, I might look like I am listening, but I am focused on what I am going to say to display my brilliance and knowledge when you stop talking.

Sometimes as I park the car, I cannot remember the drive to get there; I was that inattentive.

Even when I am standing in front of you, looking like I am present, I may not be there. My mind wanders.

That is what I do without thought or effort. Or I can choose otherwise and bring myself back to the present.

My factory default settings are set to self-possessed and wandering. If I am to be where I am, I must choose.

How do I look to God?

Tagged: #appearances, #spiritual growth, #spiritual awakening, #step 3, #step 12

Every morning I scroll through my checklist of questions,[8] often merely skimming them quickly, but occasionally one of the questions in the checklist catches my attention and brings me up short.

Such was the case with the question "How do I look to God?" I had looked at this question for years, sometimes thinking about it, sometimes glossing over it. Then one morning, I stopped; I realized that there is more to this question than I had thought.

I had always taken the question to mean that I want to "look good" in God's eyes, to follow His will, act during the day in a manner that would meet with His approval, and live in a way that He directs.

Instead of looking good in the eyes of business partners, clients, sponsees, and others, the goal was to look good in the eyes of God. To be the character that God would approve, to do the things that God would want done, to be the man that God desires.

However, that morning, I stopped and thought about this question differently. I realized that there is a second meaning to the question "How do I look to God?"

The second meaning is a reversal of the direction of the question. In the first meaning God is looking at me, and I am asking, if God is looking at me, what does He think? Is He pleased or disappointed? In the second meaning, the direction

---

[8] These checklists are shown as Worksheets on my website, the4thdimension.ca. Enjoy them and use them.

is reversed, the question focuses on me looking at God rather than God looking at me. And in that regard the question could be restated: How often and how carefully am I looking to God during the day?

Am I paying attention to Him and am I consciously aware of Him and His presence? Am I continually glancing towards Him during the day, looking for a signal as to what to do? Am I talking to Him before making critical decisions, and then listening to Him? When I am disturbed, am I looking to Him? In short, during the day, minute by minute and hour by hour, "How do I look to God?"

Now in the mornings and during the day, I think about both questions, "How do I look to God?" and "How do I look to God?"

Giving or Getting

Tagged: #inventory, #spiritual growth

B.D., a good AA friend, has a great mind that produces many keen insights which he has shared over the years.

Let me share one that has proven to be useful as a 'gut check' during the day.

He said, "In any conversation or situation, I am either giving or getting;, and when I am giving rather than getting, I feel better, and the situation or conversation almost always works out better."

If I am in the spiritual zone, I focus on what I can give rather than what I can get.

But I am not always in the spiritual zone. Often, I am not standing in the sunlight of the spirit. At those times, I focus on getting rather than giving.

There are warning signs. Flushed cheeks, rising temper, irritation — but I often ignore the warning signs and persist in getting rather than giving. I dig the hole deeper.

I can sometimes catch myself mid-step and try to change from getting to giving. I have to displace my Ego in the transition from 'getting' to 'giving;' from self-centred to other-centred. That demands mental and spiritual effort. Overcoming my self-centred focus is hard. I conceive that there are good reasons for my Ego to be involved, and I fear the consequences of displacing my precious and perfect Ego. It seems appropriate to be getting rather than giving.

After years of observation — giving rather than getting is always the better choice, even if I am mid-step.

Steps

Introduction

Steps, proposals, principles, suggestions — whatever the label, these are the actions which, counterintuitively, lead me to sobriety.

What do I mean by "counterintuitively?"

Let's look at the Steps. First, the Steps have nothing to do with the problem, stopping drinking; nowhere in the Steps does it say anything like "Then we stopped drinking." Second, alcohol is not prominent in the Steps; only the first part of Step One mentions alcohol, and it is an admission of powerlessness, not an instruction to stop. Third, Step 12, says that "The result of these steps" is "a spiritual awakening," not "We now ceased drinking." According to the end-game Step, the whole Program is all about a spiritual awakening, not about drinking.

So, I say it is counterintuitive that taking these Steps will lead to a cessation of drinking.

But the reasons don't matter. How taking the Steps lifts the desire to drink and why doing them makes us sober, is irrelevant. Bottom line, in our experience, they work. They work well: "Rarely have we seen someone fail who has thoroughly followed our path."

In an interview, long after the Big Book was written, Bill Wilson is reported to have been asked: "Would you change anything in the Big Book?"

"I would," he replied, "In How It Works I would change the word 'rarely' to 'never.'"

Based on years of experience and observation, he knew that if anyone assiduously applied these Steps to their life, they would stay sober. Experience shows that practising the Steps is a guarantee of relapse prevention for alcoholics.

This is a collection of AA GEMS about the Steps. The proposals, principles, and suggestions found in the Big Book of Alcoholics Anonymous. These are my observations, thoughts, and experience. Take what is useful and leave the rest.

12 Steps to Build a House

Tagged: #house building, #spiritual growth, #steps

"Practicing the AA program is like building a house. First, I had to pour a big, thick concrete slab on which to erect the house; that to me was the equivalent of stopping drinking. But it's pretty uncomfortable living on a concrete slab, unprotected and exposed to the heat, cold, wind and rain. So I built a room on the slab by starting to practice the Program. The first room was rickety because I wasn't used to the work. But as time passed, as I practiced the Program, I learned to build better rooms. The more I practiced, and the more I built, the more comfortable and happy was the home I now have to live in." –Bill Wilson

This is my story; I poured a foundation slab, then I lived on the slab for several years. I was not drinking, and I was succeeding in business with an impressive power drive. The same power drive applied to my service work in AA, my family life, and most other areas of my work and play.

But during that time, both I and everyone around me paid an awful price. I was an unmedicated alcoholic. The drive for success and power was on full blast. Being sober, but without a good Program, I was rarely on the spiritual beam.

Thankfully, I received a second Gift of Desperation (GoD) in sobriety. The first Gift of Desperation was the pain arising from my drinking; I became desperate enough to want to stop. The second Gift of Desperation was the carnage and bad feelings I was creating in my work, family, and AA service life. It finally penetrated my thick skull and my even thicker heart that I needed help. The second Gift of Desperation caused me to pick up the tools of the Program, the Steps, and to build my first rickety room on the concrete slab. Since then, using the tools and materials of the Program, I've been adding on to that room and building other rooms.

I've gone back and renovated some rooms. I have improved the systems in the house, looking at the ductwork, electrical work, and plumbing. I have added features like indoor plumbing, heating, and air conditioning. My home has become more comfortable and welcoming, and I can use the building tools and materials faster and better.

It has been an incredible journey. I have a happy home that is welcoming to all.

I have come to enjoy my AA home. It has taken a lot of work, but it is worth it.

I hope you are enjoying working on your AA home.

Reawakenings and Second Awakenings

Tagged: #spiritual growth, #spiritual awakening, #steps, #tools of the program

When I am asked to read How It Works at an AA Meeting, I always add two points of emphasis. I read Step 12, with added weight on A and THE: we have A spiritual awakening as THE result of these Steps.

A spiritual awakening is not a possible, or probable result of these Steps. It is the unequivocal, direct and inevitable consequence of these Steps. When we do these Steps, a spiritual awakening will occur.

Our first awakening does not have to be the only awakening that we ever have. I discovered that when I worked the Steps again, the result was another awakening. After doing the Steps again, I was more spiritually awake, more aware of God; my God consciousness had increased.

My story is a series of awakenings. Like climbing a spiral staircase, I practised the Steps in life. Each time I worked through the Steps, I completed another circle in the spiral staircase, rising higher and higher with each progression.

When I am on the spiritual beam, I bake the Steps into my life. I use them as tools to solve problems. They are recipes for successful living.

Abstinence from alcohol is a second-order effect. The endpoint of the Steps is a spiritual awakening. In my Program, I do the Steps over and over. The primary purpose of my Program is a spiritual awakening, then another, then another, and so on.

I am doing the Steps over and over again.

That has been my story.

Awakenings or Awakening

Tagged: #spiritual awakening, #step 12, #steps

My spiritual awakenings were of the educational variety. There were many lessons in the education process.

Spiritual awakenings, for me, came in a series, one after another, and they were cumulative.

My morning awakenings are like my spiritual awakenings.

I am not a morning person. Unlike my wife, who leaps out of bed, ready to take on the day, I stagger up from my sleep. There are several layers as I wake up in the morning, as I emerge from sleep to civil discourse. The alarm goes off — my first awakening; I reach over, turn it off, and hit the floor on my knees for a quick prayer: "Good morning God. I am going to need your help today." Takes two seconds — it is my second awakening. Standing up, I go into the bathroom and splash water on my face — my third awakening. I wander into the kitchen for my first coffee — another awakening, my fourth.

With each step, I am more aware and awake.

By the time I finish breakfast, I've had several awakenings. They are progressive; with each step, I am slightly more conscious and aware of the day — and they are cumulative, each one building on the last.

My spiritual awakenings were like this. When I first came into the Program, I had a first spiritual awakening. It was sufficient to get me to stop drinking, but it was just the first. Then I had another awakening; I applied the Steps to a problem in my work relations. Then a third awakening when I used the Steps to achieve victory over my smoking. Then I had a fourth awakening with sex habits. I've had awakenings over the years, dealing with different challenges and issues.

The parallels between my morning series of awakenings and my AA series of awakenings is unassailable.

With each spiritual awakening, I reach a higher level of consciousness. I'm easier to deal with. I'm more presentable to the world. With each awakening, I am more aware of my surroundings and less interested in myself.

My morning awakenings are the same. With each step in my morning routine, I am more aware and easier to get along with.

A Great Article by Bill W from the June 1958 Grapevine

Tagged: #steps, #meditation, #prayer, #awareness of god, #agnostics, #conscious awareness, #emotional sobriety, #step 11, #spiritual growth, #surrender, #in the moment, #habits, #discipline, #morning meditation, #tools of the program

This GEM is from Bill W. He is discussing Step 11. Cannot top this guy.

In this article, I'd like to turn to Step 11, for the benefit of the complete doubters, the unlucky ones who can't believe Step 11 has any real merit at all.

In lots of instances, people find their first obstacle in the phrase "God as we understand Him." The doubter is apt to say, "On the face of it, nobody can understand God. I half believe that there is a First Cause, a Something, and maybe a Somebody. But I can't get any further than this. I think people are kidding themselves when they say they can. Even if there were a Somebody, why should He bother with little me, when, in making the Cosmos run, he already has plenty to do? As for those folks who claim that God tells them where to drill for oil, or when to brush their teeth — well, they just make me tired."

Our friend is clearly one who believes in some kind of God — "God as he understands Him." But he doesn't believe any bigger concept or better feeling about God to be possible. So he looks upon meditation, prayer, and guidance as the means of self-delusion. Now, what can our hard-pressed friend do about this?

Well, he can strenuously try meditation, prayer, and guidance, just as an experiment. He can address himself to whatever God he thinks there is. Or, if he thinks there is none, he can admit — just for experimental purposes — that he might be wrong. This is all-important. As soon as he is able to take this attitude, it means that he has stopped playing God himself; his mind has opened. Like any good scientist in his laboratory, our friend can assume a theory and can make an experiment. He can pray to a "higher power" that may exist and may be willing to help and guide him. He keeps on experimenting — in this case, praying — for a long time. Again he tries to behave like the scientist, an experimenter who is never supposed to give up so long as there is a vestige of any chance of success.

As he goes along with his process of prayer, he begins to add up the results. If he persists, he will almost surely find more serenity, more tolerance, less fear and less anger. He will acquire a quiet courage, the kind that doesn't strain him. He can look at so-called failure and success for what they really are. Problems and calamity will begin to mean instruction instead of destruction. He will feel freer and saner. The idea that he may have been hypnotizing himself by auto-suggestion will become laughable. His sense of purpose and of direction will increase. His tensions and anxieties will commence to fade. His physical health is likely to improve. Wonderful and unaccountable things will start to happen. Twisted relations in his family and on the outside will unaccountably improve.

Even if few of these things happen, he will still find himself in possession of great gifts. When he has to deal with hard circumstances, he can face them and accept them. He can now accept himself and the world around him. He can do this because he now accepts a God who is All — and who loves all. When he now says, "Our Father who art in Heaven, hallowed be Thy name," our friend deeply and humbly means it. When in good meditation and thus freed from the clamours of the world, he knows that he is in God's hands, that his own destiny is really secure, here and hereafter.

A great theologian once declared, "The chief critics of prayer are those who have never really tried it enough." That's good advice — good advice I'm trying to take ever more seriously for myself. Many AA's have long been striving for a better conscious contact with God and I trust that many more of us will presently join with that wise company.

I've just finished re-reading the chapter on Step 11 in our book, "Twelve Steps and Twelve Traditions." This was written almost five years ago. I was astonished when I realized how little time I had actually been giving to my own elementary advice on meditation, prayer, and guidance — practices that I had so earnestly recommended to everybody else!

In this lack of attention I probably have plenty of company. But I do know that this is a neglect that can cause us to miss the finest experiences of life, a neglect that can seriously slacken the growth that God hopes we may achieve right here on earth, here in this great day at school, this very first of our Father's Many Mansions.

ANDY C

Spiritual Maintenance

Tagged: #awareness, #changes, #maintenance, #spiritual awakening

My sobriety is contingent on 'spiritual maintenance.' Not a spiritual cure, not a spiritual fix, just spiritual maintenance.

There is an old parlour game, "If you were a car, what kind of car would you be?"

Let me play that game.

When I started the Program, I was an old beat up piece of junk. The tires were bald; in bad weather, I would skid and slide. The engine burned more oil than gas; I was blowing plumes of blue smoke. The muffler was shot, so I was noisy and irritating. The brakes were worn out and my inability to stop or slow down caused much excitement in the parking lot. The windshield was cracked, so my vision of the world was obscured. The upholstery was ruined; the springs made me uncomfortable.

Then I started a program of maintenance on my metaphorical car. Working on each of the defects, I discovered that one repair led to another.

First, the motor, the first step in my maintenance program. I repaired it. However, once the engine was running, more power was passed to the transmission. With added power, the defects in the transmission became apparent, with much grinding and gnashing of gears. At first, I denied that there was a problem, but eventually, it seized up. So the transmission was next on the maintenance schedule. With a properly maintained engine and transmission, I had a lot more get-up-and-go, but the brakes were worn out. Not wanting to repair things too soon, I fixed the brakes only after I had plowed into a couple of other cars. With motor, transmission, and brakes maintained, I was capable of highway speeds, but now I needed new tires.

75

And so it went. Each maintenance step showed the problems that were next in need of attention, but it got better and better. With continuous maintenance and work, the wreck became a serviceable vehicle. I could get around town safely and securely. Driving was fun again.

Now sometimes there is rust or some minor wear and tear, but I have a good maintenance program. I am learning lessons in maintenance, like catching defects as soon as I see them. Early repairs are easier. If I wait, the problems get bigger, not better.

As I think of my spiritual maintenance program, the wreck of a car is my original spiritual life. I was slipping and sliding in lousy weather, creating damage and harm as I caromed around the roads of life. But I started a repair and maintenance program. The Big Book is the maintenance manual; the Steps are the tools that I use. The wrenches, drivers, pliers, and other tools are used again and again with different repairs — sex, social instincts, business relations, etc. One repair leads to another in my spiritual maintenance program.

So, I drive down the road of Happy Destiny.

It is Only Coincidental

Tagged: #awareness, #coincidence, #spiritual growth, #meetings

I'm sitting in Hilton Head getting ready to play tennis. Life couldn't be better. I went to a great Meeting last night. Nice to know that everywhere I go in North America there are lots of Meetings, each with their own style and tone, but with the same kind of people and the same message.

This was a men's Meeting. One of the fellows shared: "Over the last several years, I have practised the Steps of AA."

He paused, then continued, "I noticed that during the time I have practised the Steps, I have not been arrested or gone to jail. I have had good relations with my wife. I am on a solid career trajectory. I am generally happy, joyous, and free."

He paused... "But I am pretty sure that these are just coincidences."

As we laughed out loud, he closed by saying that, "Even though these are just coincidences, I do not want to take any chances, and I plan to continue with Meetings, Steps and sponsorship." We laughed again, with applause showing our agreement.

Thank goodness for coincidences. Thank goodness for the Program — what a wonderful, wonderful life we have so long as we follow some simple Steps.

It's not complicated, but it does require some discipline.

What Should I Expect from God?

The discussion was, "How do I do Step Three."

The question was answered with several other questions. How will He direct, manage, control, or steer me? Just what does it mean to turn my will and life over to Him and His care and protection?

What should I look for? Do I get a script to follow? Is there an instruction manual that I could read? Is there some prophet I should listen to? Will there be writing on the wall? How the hell do you accomplish Step Three?

Well, the "clear cut directions are laid out" in the last paragraph of Chapter Three of the 12 x 12. Whenever I am disturbed or making a decision, I should think about God, then wait quietly for an intuitive thought or word.

For me, with a micro-second of thought, I say, "God is in this."

This is what happens:

• My mind calms, which makes my words gentle and kind, regardless of the circumstances,

• My attitudes reset, which gives me a guideline to follow in tackling the problem, and

• My mind clears, which allows a more comprehensive perception of the situation.

All of these are instantaneous and self-reinforcing.

And it works, all of it. At least it has in my life.

Mind you, the instructions come with a caveat. In the beginning, because this tool is new and unfamiliar, we may do some odd things and things may not always work out. But it is like a new shot in tennis. The first few times you try it, weird things happen. But after a few misfires, you have it! Voila! You are an improved player.

So, accept the risks, push through what appear to be misfires, and do it.

A Gateway Step

Tagged: #spiritual awakening, #spiritual growth, #step 2, #steps

In the 50s and 60s, marijuana was described as a 'gateway drug.' Using marijuana was the gateway to stronger drugs like heroin.

Starting with the lighter and lower-impact drug, we would be exposed to the tantalizing effects of drugs in general. After using marijuana, we would desire more dangerous drugs.

A gateway drug has to be innocent and easy to use. Otherwise, it will put people off.

With marijuana, you could smoke it or eat it in brownies, easy and straightforward.

The gateway had to appear innocent. Marijuana would give you the munchies and make you laugh a lot. It seemed harmless. It had to be that way. Otherwise, it would scare the first-time users away. No sense having a gateway to invite people with a sign that says "There Be Dragons Here" or "Caution, Drug Hell Ahead."

Recently, I heard Step Two described as a gateway Step. I thought, "How cool is that?"

"We came to believe that a power greater than ourselves could restore us to sanity."

It is innocent and a gateway to spiritual life. It is simple; we come to believe. No action required; it is a mere acknowledgement. It is neither a decision nor an activity, just a coming into being.

And we don't even have to deal with God, only a Power greater than ourselves. AA's have used the group, the Program, sponsors, doorknobs, and light bulbs. It requires no actions, writings, or prayers. We only have to acknowledge that there is something greater than ourselves.

Sponsors over the decades have lured newcomers across this threshold with assurances that this is not a religious step; it is not a God thing; it is merely an acknowledgement that you are not God. "It is not that big a deal," we say.

But nested within this simple Step is a fascinating complexity. There are at least four significant insights buried in this Step.

First, it is an acknowledgement of a principle that some regard as the heart of the Program. That there is a Higher Power than ourselves. It does not demand that we acknowledge a God, only that we are not God.

Second, nested, or implicit in the Step is the suggestion that the problems we face are not outside of us, but inside. Sanity is not external but internal. The problem is not our circumstances, but how we perceive our circumstances. And a further dimension of the problem is my attitudes toward those perceptions.

Third, "the Power that is greater than ourselves" is sufficiently interested in us to be willing to take some steps or actions to restore us to a former state. This, of course, is a massive statement about the Power greater than us. It cares for us and is interested in us. Even if it is just the Program and the Fellowship, the Program and its adherents will care for you, and you are loved.

Fourth, unlike the First Step, which is an acknowledgement of our hopelessness, this is an acknowledgement of hope. There is a way out.

This innocent and straightforward Step is a gateway to the rest of the Program. With innocence, it attracts and draws you in, setting the stage for stronger Steps. You can take it easily and begin your journey.

The Tarzan Effect

Tagged: #growing up, #steps

Sometimes in our Program, we are stuck between Steps. At a recent Meeting of the Turf, a young man shared his wisdom about getting stuck between Steps. He described the 'Tarzan Effect.'

Imagine Tarzan, swinging through the jungle from vine to vine. Confident in the Higher Vine Power above, his Higher Power that holds the vines. He releases one vine and swings on the next. His Higher Vine Power is looking after the strength and positioning of the vines to carry him to some yet unseen future destination.

Imagine the Steps as vines. We swing gracefully from one Step to the next, trusting in our Higher Power. Releasing one and grabbing the next. Then the 'Tarzan Effect' occurs. We are swinging through the jungle of life, and it is glorious. We swing out far enough to grasp the next vine, but suddenly, we hesitate. Lacking confidence, we hang on to the last vine, just in case. Will our Higher Vine Power look after us? Is the new vine secure, and will it hold our weight? Will it take us somewhere dangerous? There we hang, suspended between the last and next vines, gripping both with grim determination.

Steps can be like vines. Lacking faith in our Higher Power, we hang suspended between Steps. Even at the beginning, it happens.

Often, we come into the Program, and we are stuck between drinking and the Program. When we first came into AA, we could not imagine life without booze and were afraid to trust the next vine, the Program. We did not want to let go of alcohol, which had worked to make us feel better. We wondered, can we trust this new vine to take us somewhere safe? But finally, we let go of the booze and swing forward grabbing the Program vine.

Later, after we have been sober for a while, we identify defects that stand in the way of our usefulness to others. We resist letting go of the old vine, but eventually, we learn that we can let go and swing through into the future. We decide that we can trust our Higher Vine Power, the Higher Step Power.

So, when we tell our sponsees to "let go," we can add, "You are suffering from the Tarzan effect. Let go of the last vine and swing through on the next. The worst case is that you swing back like a pendulum, to where you started. The best case is that you move forward through the jungle to catch up with Jane."

Let Go and trust in the Higher Vine Power.

Practicing Step 11, by Bill Wilson

Tagged: #Bill Wilson, #meditation, #spiritual growth, #step 11, #steps

This GEM is a powerful message from Bill W. In his own words:

One Man's View*

WHEN IT COMES TO THE PRACTICE of AA's Step 11 — "Sought through prayer and meditation to improve our conscious contact with God as we understood Him, praying only for knowledge of His will for us and the power to carry that out" — I'm sure I am still very much in the beginner's class; I'm almost a case of arrested development.

Around me I see many people who make a far better job of relating themselves to God than I do. Certainly it mustn't be said I haven't made any progress at all over the years; I simply confess that I haven't made the progress that I might have made, my opportunities being what they have been, and still are.

My twenty-fourth AA anniversary is just ahead; I haven't had a drink in all this time. In fact, I've scarcely been tempted at all. This is some evidence that I must have taken and ever since maintained Step One: "We admitted we were powerless over alcohol, that our lives had become unmanageable." Step One was easy for me.

Then, at the very beginning, I was fortunate enough to receive a tremendous spiritual awakening and was instantly "made conscious of the presence of God" and "restored to sanity" — at least so far as alcohol is concerned. Therefore, I've had no difficulty with AA's Step Two because, in my case, its content was an outright gift. Step Four and Step Five, dealing with self-survey and confession of one's defects, have not been overly difficult, either.

Of course, my self-analysis has frequently been faulty. Sometimes I've failed to share my defects with the right people; at other times, I've confessed their defects, rather than my own; and at still other times, my confession of defects has been more in the nature of loud complaints about my circumstances and my problems.

Nevertheless, I think I've usually been able to make a fairly thorough and searching job of finding and admitting my personal defects. So far as I know, there isn't at this moment a single defect or current problem of mine which hasn't been discussed with my close advisers. Yet this pretty well-ventilated condition is nothing for self-congratulation. Long ago I was lucky enough to see that I'd have to keep up my self-analysis or else blow my top completely. Though driven by stark necessity, this continuous self-revelation—to myself and to others—was rough medicine to take. But years of repetition has made this job far easier. Step Nine, making restitution for harms done, has fallen into much the same bracket.

In Step 12 —carrying the AA message to others—I've found little else than great joy. We alkies are folks of action and I'm no exception. When action pays off as it does in AA, it's small wonder that Step 12 is the most popular and, for most of us, the easiest one of all.

This little sketch of my own "pilgrim's progress" is offered to illustrate where I, and maybe lots of other AA's, have still been missing something of top importance. Through lack of disciplined attention and sometimes through lack of the right kind of faith, many of us keep ourselves year after year in rather easy a spiritual kindergarten I've just described. But almost inevitably we become dissatisfied; we have to admit we have hit an uncomfortable and maybe a very painful sticking point.

Twelfth-Stepping, talking at meetings, recitals of drinking histories, confession of our defects and what progress we have made with them no longer provide us with the released and abundant life. Our lack of growth is often revealed by an unexpected calamity or a big emotional upset. Perhaps we hit the financial jackpot and are surprised that this solves almost nothing that we are still bored and miserable, notwithstanding.

As we usually don't get drunk on these occasions, our bright-eyed friends tell us how well we are doing.

But inside, we know better. We know we aren't doing well enough. We still can't handle life, as life is. There must be a serious flaw somewhere in our spiritual practice and development.

What then, is it?

The chances are better than even that we shall locate our trouble in our misunderstanding or neglect of AA's Step 11 — prayer, meditation and the guidance of God. The other Steps can keep most of us sober and somehow functioning. But Step 11 can keep us growing, if we try hard and work at it continually. If we expend even five percent of the time on Step 11 that we habitually (and rightly) lavish on Step 12, the results can be wonderfully far-reaching. That is an almost uniform experience of those who constantly practice Step 11.

Getting Out of the Rooms

Tagged: #program, #step 9, #steps

I heard a great speaker last week.

There were several noteworthy points, but one, in particular, leapt onto my notebook, "When we hit the ninth Step, we get out of the Rooms, and our Program meets the real world for the first time."

What an excellent observation. When we hit the ninth Step, for the first time, we are dealing with a non-Program person, in a non-Program conversation, outside of the Rooms. It is 'Showtime' in the real world for our Program and our new way of life.

There were and are amends that I make to other AA's, but most of my amends have been with Normies, non-AA's.

Caution and care are the watchwords.

We are in the real world. We are in our old environment but with a new way of approaching it. Careful thought, prayer, and preparation are highly recommended, with an emphasis on prayer.

The amend might include a conversation about the Program, and its values and our journey. Remember, you are dealing with someone who does not know the jargon of AA, does not know the rules and conventions of AA, and probably does not care. So, we have to watch our language.

The amend might be with someone who still thinks badly of us. We might not be welcomed with open arms. Again, prayer and restraint of pen and tongue are essential Program virtues to keep in mind.

I have some time in the Program, but life continues. I still screw up and have to make amends. Thus, I am still making amends with Normies, doing my part to make the relationships right. My Program continues to meet the outside world.

And even now, after many years, it is good to remind myself that the Normies I am dealing with don't speak our AA jargon. If I am making an amend, there can be issues. "Good to see you, Andy" might not be the greeting I receive. Great care is still to be taken. And prayer is relevant, as is a detailed planning session with my sponsor.

Amends are the first and full contact of our Program with the real world.

Mental Real Estate

Tagged: #forgiveness, #freedom, #resentments, #spiritual growth, #step 4

Just writing down the names of people who irritate me clears away mental real estate. The names are no longer in my mind; they are on the paper.

In the Big Book fourth Step instructions for an inventory, the first thing to do is write a 'Grudge List' of people that have irritated me, made me angry, harmed me, bothered me, or were a source of resentment. For the eighth Step, I write another list of names.

In both cases, writing the names starts a process. I clear the real estate in my mind by writing the names.

These people were occupying space in my mind. They each had a footprint in my mentality. By writing their names down on paper, they were objectified. After that, they are on paper, not in my mind.

By doing nothing more than writing the names down, I have begun the process of release and redemption. I have freed that mental space for more productive uses.

Simple lists of names on paper. Such is the genius of the Program.

Self-Will / Ego

Introduction

In the Program, we identify self-will as the central problem in our lives. A word search of 'self-will' in the Big Book reveals many references, including:

• "An alcoholic is an extreme example of self-will run riot, though he usually doesn't think so."

• "Any life run on self-will can hardly be a success."

• "Self-will has blocked you off from Him."

• "The debris which has accumulated out of our effort to live on self-will and run the show ourselves…"

• "We ask especially for freedom from self-will."

Self-will is a problem, and problems need to be solved.

For me, the most challenging part of this problem, the problem of self-will, is the persistence of my Ego. It seems that I cannot ever think enough about 'me.' I make decisions based on what I want, what I think is right, what I think will make me feel good. I, I, I and me, me, me. Self-centred thinking.

The problem of Ego and self-centred thinking is a mental problem. It is not a physical phenomenon; it is mental. It is a habit of thought. Since it is thinking about myself that causes the problems; I have to eliminate, or at least reduce, self and Ego from my thinking.

But I cannot erase thoughts. I cannot stop thinking about something. Imagine a strawberry milkshake on a hot day. Got it in your mind's eye? Good. Now stop thinking about that strawberry milkshake. Stop thinking about the cold, strawberry flavour. Stop thinking about the pink colour and great taste.

You cannot stop thinking about the strawberry milkshake.

Now imagine a chocolate sundae. Think about the ice cream, the fudge, nuts and a cherry on top.

The strawberry milkshake has vanished, replaced by the thought of a chocolate sundae. I cannot stop thinking about things, but I can replace the idea of things. Concentrating on stopping thinking about something means focusing on that very thing. I have to replace one thought with another thought.

Thinking about myself is the same. I cannot stop thinking about my opinions, desires, thoughts and interests. I cannot stop thinking about myself; I have to replace those thoughts of self with something else. Thinking about God is a great alternative, a great replacement. But any Power greater than myself will do. I must ask myself, "what does my Higher Power think, desire, or want?"

This idea of what we are thinking about is crucial. As long as the thoughts of Ego and self-sufficiency are present, a Higher Power cannot be present. God cannot, or will not, argue with us on this point. If we want to assert our will and let our Ego dominate our thoughts, He will back away immediately. He will leave us alone.

At least that is my experience.

No external force will trigger the solution to the problem. We have to *will* the answer. We have to desire God enough to invite Him into our lives.

These GEMs focus on Ego and self-will and how we deal with this problem.

Came Hard and Remained Firm

Tagged: #faith, #God as I understood Him, #restless irritable and discontented, #spiritual awakening, #spiritual experiences

In my Program, spiritual growth has come hard but remains firm; in contrast with my old ways of spiritual growth, characterized by easy come, easy go.

All the memories of my youth are coloured with shades of grey unease and deep discontent, even though I had a wonderful childhood and adolescence.

My first solution to relieve the greyness was discovered at an Evangelical Rally (an old-fashioned revival) at our church when I gave my life to Christ. My idea of how God would work in my life was simple; it was one and done. With the acceptance of my Saviour, publicly announced, the conversion was complete. I was to be transformed, in the twinkling of an eye, made perfect, with all my sins forgiven. Nothing more was required. This conversion experience was the first of four times that I gave my life to Him. The expression 'Indian Giver' is no longer politically correct, but that is what I was. Four times I gave my life to Him, and four times I took it back. The spiritual experiences did not last, but they did, temporarily, solve the sense of unease and discontent. I quickly lost each surge of joy and completeness, with the assistance of drugs, then alcohol.

The spiritual flash came easy then went away easy.

Then I discovered booze; this was a reliable solution. It dissolved my unease and discontent. Though the effect was temporary, it could be renewed with another drink.

It would have been a perfect solution, but there was a problem, I had a physical allergy; I did not stop when the sense of unease and discontent disappeared. With thoughtless momentum, I would proceed past the point of ease and contentment, to alcohol-induced oblivion. I always overshot the mark.

I came to AA, which to my initial horror, involved a spiritual solution. At first, I thought it was going to be another religious conversion experience, but this time was different. In the Program, I had to surrender my old ideas of frothy religious conversion experiences being a one and done solution. I had to replace my former thoughts of God and how He was going to work in my life, with new ideas of God and how He would work in my life.

What were the new ideas that I found when I arrived in AA? The new ideas were the disciplines of the Steps. These principles, practised in all my affairs, led to a sturdy and more permanent spiritual growth.

This new process was not 'easy come.' It took numerous inventories, fifth Step confessional conversations and much striving to improve my character by aligning my will with God's. It involved many hours of working the Program in Meetings, with newcomers, answering crisis phone calls and other service work. It included reading, study, prayer, and meditation. But the results were worth it; the spiritual growth lasted longer; it remained firm.

The old ways: easy come and easy go.

The new ways: hard come and hard go.

Good Start to the Day

Tagged: #in the moment, #present

A drunk looked up from the gutter to see a 'swell' entering an exclusive hotel, dressed in a smart suit with a gorgeous babe on his arm and a silk scarf around his neck.

He muttered to himself "there, but for me, go I."[9]

Getting out of my own way is a struggle.

For me, it starts in the morning, in my preparation for the day. I review the day ahead. The simple and practical form of meditation that Bill W. suggests in our Big Book.

I look at my calendar and imagine the meetings, phone calls, and conversations that are ahead, thinking about each one. I visualize each one, working through possible problems and benefits, being mindful of God during this process.

It just takes a minute and yields excellent results.

Recently, I spoke with L.S. from the Turf. He had been reading Dr. Bob and the Good Old-Timers, and he noticed that "back in the old days of AA, morning preparation for the day was more important than Meetings."

I think that he is right. My morning preparation is more important than Meetings. (Interesting observation, when I am diligent in my morning preparation, I often feel like a Meeting. I have the time and energy to attend AA Meetings, and be entirely in the moment at those Meetings.)

A morning meditation sets the day up, like a golf ball on a tee. I am set up for a great drive. I can still shank or slice the ball

---

[9] Full credit to R.P. of the Elbow Park group in Calgary. Hope that he is still around.

during the day, but correctly set up, my chances of success improve.

Do I Need an Audience?

Happy, Joyous & Free: The Lighter Side of Sobriety has some great GEMs.

One is the difference between Ego and Self Esteem: "Self Esteem does not require an audience, while Ego wants a loud and enthusiastic crowd."

This simple insight has dominated my thinking all week.

All too often, I crave an audience. My Ego, which is usually running both my thinking and my life, demands an audience, applause, and glorification. When the audience is not there and applauding loudly, I become restless, irritated, and discontented.

But when I am in the spiritual zone and aware of my inner, authentic and true self, the self that lives in a place of self-esteem, I don't need an audience.

Well, maybe just a small audience; the sunlight of the spirit. I need an audience of one. That one is God, and may I find Him now.

Anger and Perfectionism

Tagged: #anger, #growth, #pride, #self-centered

There were two topics for discussion at the Meeting: anger and perfection. Perhaps they are not separate topics; maybe they are one phenomenon.

In the past, I had to feel good at all times; I had to look perfect. If these conditions were not met, I became angry.

I had to find the 'causes and conditions' of this problem and attack it at its roots. I had to find the 'exact nature' of the problem.

The exact nature of the defect was more profound than the lack of control of my temper. The exact nature of the anger, the source of my anger, was a mental state that preceded the temper tantrum or feeling of anger; I thought I was a demigod who could make life perfect.

After thorough inventories and conversations with my spiritual coach, I saw the exact nature of the problem, the mental state that was the precursor to anger; I thought that I was a god. Not the big God, who created and governed the universe, just a small god, responsible for managing my part of the world. And this minor deity demanded perfection in his corner of the world.

This was a problem of Ego and pride. A level of pride and Ego that allowed me to think I could manage the world around me.

But pride and Ego were not enough to manage the world around me; I could not control life and make it perfect. Reality did not make me feel happy all the time. And if reality was not making me happy, I faced an existential threat. My lack of happiness meant that I was not God, and that was unacceptable. Rather than accept reality as it was, I exploded in rage.

Identifying the cause and condition of my anger helped. Courtroom lawyers say, "A question asked well is half answered." Similarly, "A defect well-named is half-resolved." I had now identified the nature of the wrong.

How could this be solved? I could solve it by thinking more about the Big God, my Higher Power, and deferring to Him during the day, in small and large questions, to follow His direction during the day. To pause and ask for guidance with an awareness of His presence.

When I am in the zone, it works; at least it has for me.

* I commend to one and all Ernst Kurtz's book, *Not God*.

Unconscious Contact with God

Tagged: #conscious awareness, #emotional sobriety, #growth, #spiritual awakening, #spiritual growth, #step 11

Step 11 of our Program is definite. We are to improve our conscious contact with God.

When I was younger in the Program, I read Step 11 and heard it at every Meeting but gave only passing regard to the word "conscious." But it now looms large in my life. Bill did not suggest "sub-conscious" or "unconscious" contact with God, he suggested, "conscious" contact. I see now that for many years, I had an "unconscious" rather than a "conscious" contact with God. Ironically, I became conscious of conscious.

And having conscious contact with God seems to be a necessary condition for the maintenance of a spiritual life. My pre-Program spiritual life included many emotional born-again spiritual awakenings. Regrettably, each of these experiences evaporated, requiring another. Bill, in the Big Book, describes these sudden emotional conversion experiences as "Frothy."

Looking back, I see that these pre-Program spiritual experiences went away because I assumed it was 'one and done.' I suppose that this assumption came from the massive emotional impact of these conversion experiences. These religious conversions were so great I thought that God would penetrate my mind and look after things, without any effort on my part. However, with only an unconscious or sub-conscious contact with God, my spiritual awakening would pass away.

Program life is different. It demands that I work with prayer and meditation on my conscious contact with God. With the AA Program, and in particular Step 11 and the suggestions of both prayer and meditation aimed at an improved conscious connection with God, my spiritual awakening is on a livelier footing; less likely to pass away.

Upsettable with Myself

Tagged: #anger, #God as I understood Him, #inventory, #spiritual awakening, #step 5

An AA speaker recently recalled talking with a sponsee. The sponsee was going through a difficult time; he was upset.

"Why am I upset?" he complained bitterly.

The sponsor replied: "You are upset because you are upsettable."

I could see the sponsee rolling his eyes, thinking, "What good is this advice?, I need a new sponsor, someone more sensitive to my feelings."

But it is a great response. When I am upset, an excellent first step is to ask, "Why am I upsettable?"

If something internal has caused the upset, it is a great opening question.

If something external to me has caused it, I might be able to remove the cause of my being upset. But even then, it is useful to look inward and ask why it would upset me, rather than motivate me to take some constructive and loving action. If I cannot remove the cause of my being upset, I have to explore the internal condition that made me upsettable.

Any way you look at it, "Why am I upsettable?" is a good question.

By asking this question, I can ignore the apparent cause and deal with the underlying condition. The underlying condition is between my ears, not in my circumstances. The problem is a lack of cleanliness, or sanity, in my thinking.

My experience shows that I am usually upsettable because I am focused on myself. That is the lack of sanity in my thinking. When I am self-centred, I am prone to becoming up-settable.

The symptoms often include taking my opinions seriously, negatively judging a situation or a person, thinking that I am something special — generally preoccupied with my views and myself.

I am upsettable because I am focused on myself. When I turn and focus on awareness of God, then I am not upsettable. Who could get upset when God is in charge of the outcomes?

Moreover, if I orient my mind to service to those around me, and focus on someone else, then I care more about you than me. I become un-upsettable

So if I am upset, it is because I was upsettable.

Dry Spells

Tagged: #awareness, #step 10, #step 11

In my sobriety, I have had, periods of spiritual dryness — times when I felt out of touch with God.

Years ago, I shared this with my sponsor. He suggested I read a Psalm a day. Following his instructions as I always did, I read a Psalm every day. I thought that he was pointing me to something that would get me thinking about spiritual matters. That might have been his intention, but there was more. After about 20 days, I discerned a pattern.

Psalm writers use expressions like: "God, why have you forsaken me," "God, I thirst for you," "God, I yearn for you," and "God, I am starved for you." References to dryness and abandonment in their spiritual lives. The frequency of these expressions is startling.

I was greatly comforted by this. If the spiritual heavyweights of the Old Testament had spiritual dry periods, then I can have them too. I could give myself a break.

And the lesson did not end there. I also realized that when the Psalm writers had a bad stretch, they kept going, performing the habits of spiritual life, until they reconnected with God. When you are going through a spiritual dry spell, keep up the habits of prayer and meditation. Remember the old military expression: "When you are going through the valley of the shadow of death, the worst thing you can do is stop."

Just keep going. Persistence is a cardinal virtue in a spiritual life.

The Safe Cracker and the Businessman

Tagged: #self-centered, #step 5

Self-centred thinking is a big part of our problem. In the Big Book, Bill W. gives the five biggest and baddest examples of self-centred people that he can imagine. He identifies five egregious examples, so it behooves us to spend some time considering them.

To remind you, they are:

1. The businessman, lolling on the beach complaining about the state of the world.

2. The politician, looking for utopia.

3. The preacher, preaching the one right way.

4. The safecracker, robbing rich people only.

5. The raving alcoholic, who has destroyed everything.

These are Bill's examples of the root cause of all of our problems, self-centred thinking and actions.

But what the heck? Are these the worst examples he could list?

The alcoholic and the safecracker are great examples of behaviours causing damage and harm, but what about the other three, the businessman, politician, and preacher? What is so harmful about these guys?

The businessman, politician, and preacher don't cause apparent harm and wreckage. Certainly not like the safecracker and the alcoholic. But the attitudes of the businessman, politician, and preacher are identical to the self-centred perceptions and attitudes held by the safecracker and alcoholic, and in the end, they have the same capacity for damage.

The seeds of judgment are planted when the businessman complains that the state of the nation is not as he would have it. The seeds of intolerance are planted by the politician convinced that he is right, and his is the only right way. The seeds of destruction are planted by the preacher arguing for utopia if only people would follow his path.

These seeds of judgment, intolerance, and destruction can lie dormant for a time; the effect is not immediate, but they sprout and grow into resentments, fears, and anger.

I suffered from the self-centred attitudes and perceptions of the businessman, politician, and preacher. I was complaining and judging because the world was not unfolding in a manner that made me feel good. I was judging and condemning.

My judgmental attitudes did not have immediate consequences, but they inevitably led to anger, frustration, irritation, and difficulties. They affected my marriage because I was judgmental and opinionated. They touched my business relationships because I was convinced mine was the only way. They influenced my political activities, putting blinkers on what I thought was right and proper and excluding all other views.

The self-centred mental seeds of judgment sprouted and grew to actual problems and harms.

With the three apparent innocents, the businessman, politician, and preacher, Bill was telling us, if we plant the seeds of self-centred attitudes and perceptions, we will reap the harvest.

A Sidewise Glance

Tagged: #fear, #complications, #steps

A friend shared at a recent Meeting that he can feel fear if someone looks at him sidewise. Just a sidewise glance from a stranger, and he can feel a sense of being wronged, and that can grow into a sense of being hurt. This, in turn, can mature to a full-blown feeling of anger and shame.

I have experienced the same phenomenon.

With a mere glance, we have not been physically touched. The person might not even be aware that he is looking askance, but we react. This is not a fear that comes from a threat. It is not like rustling in the brush stimulating our prehistoric survival mechanism of fear, nor a lit fuse of a stick of dynamite with the anticipated explosion to come, nor the fear of a spider that might bite.

The feelings that my friend described, which I feel all too frequently, come from a projection of future feelings of embarrassment or inadequacy; these fears are only a mental reality. It is all in my head.

Once again, I find that preoccupation with myself leads to fears, insecurities, and complications.

Inventories and Beyond

Introduction

If spiritual awakenings are the goal, removal of defects is the process.

But a defect has to be seen and identified before it can be removed.

In my experience, the fourth Step and tenth Step processes, written inventories, the processes by which I start to identify my defects, are critical. It is by doing inventories that we can begin to see and know our defects of character and shortcomings. The inventories are the stories of our defects, the anecdotes of our sins. It is the beginning of the process. The fifth Step completes it.

The fifth Step process has two parts: confession and conversation. Confession to release the energy of secrets, and conversation to refine the defects identified, distilling them to arrive at the exact nature of the wrongs. After sharing and discussing the defects with a good coach, I walk away with a clear identification of the exact nature of the underlying problem that was manifested in all the anecdotes of my defects.

I have not been able to stumble along and have God remove defects which are unnamed. An unfocused general sense of hope that my character will be improved is not a method that has worked for me. In my experience, God works with flaws that I can see and name. Inventories and confessional conversations are essential to my Program. I take a lot of inventories, both moral and personal, with both global scope and specific focus.

These GEMS are focused on the identification of the exact nature of my defects — inventories and confessional conversations, a critical feature of my recovery landscape.

Ashamed

Tagged: #shame, #inventory, #daily habits, #ego, #feelings, #self centred

I am ashamed to admit this story, but it is true.

One night, during my nightly bedtime inventory, I wrote a sponsee's name in my Grudge List. He and I had talked that day. I left the conversation with a degree of irritation. I had not even concluded our session with a word of prayer as I usually do.

In my inventory that night, I reviewed the session. I wrote out the points that bothered me. I was horrified when my pencil traced out the words "He disagreed with me."

To my shame, I realized I was upset because he expressed disagreement with something I had said.

My arrogance, the self-centred pride and intellectual preening, was astounding.

OMG, how massive an Ego to do I have?

One that is large enough to require daily inventories.

The Exact Nature

Tagged: #inventory, #emotional sobriety, #spiritual growth, #annual, #step 10, #step 5, #self-centered, #growing up, #working the steps

When I do inventories, I tell my stories of wrongs and defects. Each anecdote is a manifestation of the underlying nature of the wrong. A theme or principle is operating in my life that is causing the manifestation, and this is what I am looking for — the themes or principles, the exact nature.

There may be hundreds of stories that are manifestations of the same problem; identifying the exact nature of the wrong is a process of taking all of these stories and distilling them into the principles that are causing the behaviours. I review the many manifestations of the wrong and boil them down until I am left with the theme or underlying cause.

By way of example, imagine that you are working with a sponsee who admits in his fifth Step with you that he has shoplifted hundreds of times. Sometimes, he was caught and brought to court. Often, he was not. As you talk with him, an exact nature of a defect is revealed: he is a kleptomaniac. This distillation allows him to identify the defect and its nature better. With God's help, he can control this defect.

The anecdotes revealed the exact nature of the wrong. We need the exact *nature* of the wrongs, not the exact *details* of the wrongs.

With God's help, he can pray to be relieved of the obsession to shoplift. God can help him control his kleptomania and resist shoplifting.

Not the Same Old, Same Old

Tagged: #inventory, #step 10, #discipline, #habits, #subsequent awakenings, #naming defects, #working the steps

In annual inventories, old stories can come back to my mind, but they are not the same old, same old. Deeper insights can be obtained.

Imagine a sponsee, the same one we mentioned in the last GEM. He told you the story of 300 episodes of shoplifting. He was a kleptomaniac.

Five years later, you are still working with him. In his annual inventory, these shoplifting incidents come to his mind again, even though they have been resolved and amends have been made. He paid the shopkeepers, apologized to the police and even wrote a letter to the judges.

But there they are again; they come into his mind as he writes his annual inventory.

As you work with him, you both see a deeper problem, a deeper theme that underlies the stories of shoplifting. As you talk, he begins to see that there was a more subtle force at work: entitlement. He thinks back and recalls that as he stole the goods, lifting them from the shelf, he had a profound feeling of entitlement. He felt utterly entitled to remove those items from the store shelf.

Together you take a deeper dive into the root of the problem, and entitlement is the new, more profound, exact nature identified.

He had asked for his kleptomania to be removed and now, he and his Higher Power can work on removal of this deep sense of entitlement.

And this sense of entitlement was not limited to shoplifting. In his fifth Step confessional conversation, you and he realize that in all areas of his life he felt 'entitled' and that this deep sense of entitlement was a direct cause of many of the problems that still plague him. With this recognition, he begins working, with prayer and meditation, to have this defect removed, which in turn draws him closer to his Higher Power.

With distance and maturity, I can see the more exact nature of the defects, but only if I persist in regular inventories.

Patterns Revealed, Secrets Denied

Tagged: #step 5, #step 10, #inventory, #habits, #discipline, #removing defects, #working the steps

As an investor, I learned the importance of inventories. Management cannot run a business without accurate and precise knowledge of their stock.

In business, surprises come out of inventories: things that were not seen before, hidden patterns.

I was called in to help prepare a company for sale; we did a full inventory. We discovered the inventory was so large that it equalled one year's gross sales. There was a problem. What was going on? When we met and discussed this problem, we realized that management was afraid of telling a customer that they might have to wait for a part, even the most exotic parts. This fear led to overstocking. A good supply of even the most unusual parts had to be kept on hand. That made the company less valuable. But we did not see it until we had done a detailed inventory.

Another story. A company serviced and installed heavy machinery. They had a considerable supply of valuable specialty cement. It was precious, and when it was needed, it was required immediately. But some of the bags were 15 years old. Something was wrong. It turns out that customers had found other solutions, and this company was holding an inventory of this unique product for their legacy installs. Management knew about the latest solutions and knew that the special cement was not needed as much. Until they saw the inventory numbers and explored the exact nature of the inventory buildup, they had not seen the patterns in the changed business model. What used to be good stock had become bad stock.

So, inventories can be surprising. They show patterns that we deny or don't perceive.

That was my story. Starting my first personal inventory, I put pen to paper and got started. I did some work on it every day for a few weeks. One day I wrote a sentence, and I stopped. I thought, "I have written this sentence before." Sure enough, that was the fifth time that I had written the same sentence in just a few pages.

But here was the surprise: If you had asked me before I started this inventory "Does this phrase reflect your attitudes and beliefs?" I would have denied it. I would have protested enthusiastically. I would have denied that I was thinking that way, for the sentiment was offensive and did not reflect my identity as a young, urbane, cosmopolitan lawyer. But there was the offending phrase, in my handwriting. It pointed to outmoded thinking and attitudes. A hidden pattern was revealed in my written inventory. Surprise!

Almost every time I have done an inventory, I have found a surprise. I look forward to it now, and it is something new for God to work on.

Inventories Get Easier

Tagged: #step 5, #step 10, #inventory, #discipline, #habits, #removing defects, #working the steps

Any task becomes easier with practice and repetition.

My wife and I owned a large home, great for entertaining. We regularly hosted large dinner parties for clients and friends. They were fun to organize, and we greatly enjoyed them.

In the parties, there was a lesson to be learned. The first parties were harder to organize than the later. When we first hosted a dinner party, we had to think about everything. The dishes and cutlery had to be found. The silver was not often used, so it had to be polished. We had to think carefully about the menu.

But as we hosted more and more dinner parties, they became easier and easier. We did not have to think as much because so many of the Steps had been habituated. With practice and repetition, we remembered where things were stored and how things came together. Menus, once tried and tested, could be repeated. For us as hosts, the evenings became more comfortable and more relaxed.

And the evenings, for us, were not just more relaxed, they became better. We found that with the more relaxed setup and preparation, familiar through repetition, we had time and energy to focus on extras. I started thinking about guest seating more carefully, name tags to mark seating at the table, different napkins, etc. The small touches made the evening special.

Repetition made hosting the dinners easier and more comfortable; and also made them better.

So too with inventories. The more I do them, the easier they get. With repeated inventories under my belt, I became used to the work and knew what to expect. With practice, they became better. I could focus on deeper issues and see more clearly the underlying themes and principles that governed my life, identifying defects with greater exactitude.

So do them. Lots of them. Do the best you can each time. Keep doing them, they get more comfortable and easier with each turn of the wheel.[10]

·

---

[10] I do a yearly inventory. This is in addition to my other inventories, including spot inventories on issues that come up (lousy temper, irritations, etc.), inventories on domains in my life (family, business, sex conduct, sports, etc.), inventories on specific targets (CRA, wife, business partners, etc.), and inventories about situations (business failures, business successes, interpersonal problems, etc.)

Inventory taking

Tagged: #annual, #habits, #inventory, #spiritual awakening, #spiritual experiences, #spiritual growth, #step 10, #steps

As Bill Wilson writes in the Big Book:

"A business which takes no regular inventory usually goes broke. Taking a commercial inventory is a fact-finding and fact-facing process. ... We did exactly the same thing with our lives. We took stock honestly. First, we searched out the flaws in our make-up which caused our failure."

Businesses conduct annual inventories, so I decided to do a yearly businesslike inventory. November 3rd is my AA birthday. It seemed to me that was as good a date as any to conduct an annual inventory.

The process reveals patterns. I discover patterns about myself that I hitherto denied. Every time I conduct this annual process, I have found new patterns. Pen and paper reveal all; I cannot bullshit the paper.

And each year, I find two or three significant defects. These are the defects that my Higher Power can work on during the year. I am convinced that God works with these inventories to steer me to the flaws which He sees are causing problems.

These annual inventories have been an excellent process for me. I now believe God has used my annual inventory processes to help me identify, and then with His help, deal with defects. As a result, I deal with them in a manner and in a time that God sees fit.

As I sometimes say, "If you want what I have, you have to be a bit obsessive." This annual process, followed by analysis and synthesis, may not be for everybody, but it sure works for me.

*Resentment: a feeling of (bitter) indignation resulting from perceived or actual harm. In building my Grudge List, I include people, institutions, and principles, who are irritating, off-putting, or just difficult.

Fearful and Shameful Inventory

Tagged: #dependency on the opinion of others, #discipline, #habits, #inventory, #need for praise, #small things, #step 4

Some of my inventories are not so much to be feared as to be embarrassed.

In my inventories, there was no murder or theft, but there was a surplus of Ego.

Small things would set me off. People made me angry by failing to bow to me and acknowledge how perfect I was. The world was not treating me with the respect I was due. The world was looking at me the wrong way.

I could have a conversation at work in the afternoon; if I were not credited with brilliance and praised for the work that I had done, I would leave the conversation with a general sense of unease. If I were not focused on God consciousness, this small seed of discomfort would find good soil in my soul. Rich and dark, perfect gardening soil, moist with nutrients and potential. The seed might lie for a bit as I went through the day, then later sprout and take root, with a familiar sense of impending doom (my favourite pride manifestation). Finally, much later in the day, it would grow, ready to bear fruit. I might be with my wife at that time, so she would receive the harvest of anger and resentment with my snarly and difficult attitude.

However, I can catch the seed of discomfort and pride before it sprouts, grows, and bears fruit. It might show up in my nightly review and checklist, my daily Step Ten. In the cold light of pen and paper, I can see that my sour evening mood is the conscious and emotional manifestation of my afternoon need for praise and honour. Thank God for that simple discipline.

If people could see my inventories, their first reactions might not be horror, but laughter. They would be amused at the size of my Ego and my overly sensitive nature. My fear of the fourth Step was not the possibility of jail; instead, it was the possibility of my sponsor collapsing in laughter at the self-possessed triviality of many of my reactions to life.

Deeper Over Time

Tagged: #discipline, #habits, #inventory, #spiritual awakening, #step 4

Fred, the Big Book accountant, said, "... the program (taking the Steps) of action, though entirely sensible, was pretty drastic. It meant I would have to throw several lifelong conceptions out of the window." (page 42, the Big Book)

For several early years in my sobriety, I did not take any Steps or do any actions that were "drastic." And I did not throw any "lifelong conceptions" out the window. There were only minor adjustments to my actions; small changes to some lightly-held beliefs. I might have thrown a few casual conceptions out the window, but nothing serious.

Going to Meetings and service work kept me sober. That was sufficient to remove the compulsion to drink. Dry, but a white-knuckle time.

My attitudes remained unchanged; lifelong conceptions, unchanged; lousy temper, perfectionism, self-will, and a brutal need to win — all unchanged. As time passed, both the discomfort I experienced and the discomfort I imposed on people around me increased.

To relieve the discomfort, I had to change. I had to take actions that were more drastic and more serious. I had some lifelong conceptions that were causing problems.

First, a renewed fourth Step. My early Step Four reviews were not 'searching and fearless.' Instead, they were 'casual and shallow.' Enough at that time, but for real change, a deeper dive was needed. I came to see that unless I was experiencing a degree of fear in doing a fourth Step, I could not claim 'fearless' and unless I found something new, I could not claim 'searching.'

The joy that I experienced with more advanced Step Four reviews was a positive reinforcement to tackle the other Steps with a similar attitude. I commenced a habit of doing the Steps over and over, with new actions that were drastic and I found more lifelong preconceptions that I could throw out the window.

Applying the inventory process, to new situations or difficulties, I experienced the identification, then removal of defects, lifted, again and again — each time, more profound than the last.

So, my first pass on the Steps, my inventory process was shallow but adequate. Subsequent work was more in-depth. For me, that has been the practical meaning of "Working the Steps."

Habits of Meditation

Tagged: #daily checklist, #habits, #morning checklist, #morning meditation, #working the steps, #steps

I knew AA's were the experts in stopping drinking, and I came for help. However, the help included changing my habits of living.

In particular, Step 11; the idea of a morning planning session, "where we review the day ahead" preparing for meetings and calls. This meditation[11] allows me to set up my day mentally and spiritually. Setting myself up for the day enables me to enter situations with the right attitudes; moreover, with the preparation for the expected problems, I react better to any unexpected events.

It puts me in the same frame of mind as my non-alcoholic wife. As she enters meetings of boards and committees, she naturally gravitates to feelings such as "These are good people," "These are people I should pay attention to," and "These people have their own needs and prerogatives, and I should acknowledge them."

Me, not so much. Unprepared, I gravitate to the opposite. Attitudes like: "These people should acknowledge my leadership," "these people are here to listen to me," and "These people should be grateful to know me."

But if, in my morning meditation, I think about a meeting or conversation that is planned for later that day, and I prepare with short notes in my calendar, these attitudes can be amended.

---

[11] Interestingly, an old meaning, found in a 1930s vintage dictionary, for the word 'meditation' includes strategic planning and business planning. A general in the army meditates on his war plan. A businessman meditates on his business plan.

With forethought, I can approach the meeting or conversation with the attitudes that my wife instinctively brings into these situations. This idea of a morning planning session, a morning meditation on the day, sets me up and makes my day better.

It is the actions. The actions of morning meditation change my thinking. Sure works for me.

Four Columns of Insight

Tagged: #annual, #inventory, #step 4, #step 10

My reading of the Big Book shows several approaches to inventories. Over the years, I have found the four-column method to be the best and most revealing.

I start with column #1, the Grudge List; the names that made me angry, sore, burned up or bugged me. The list includes all the relationships that are not "just right." The relationships that are somehow out of focus or out of kilter. I relax and write down the names that come to mind and let things flow. I don't try to think about *why* the name might occur to me.

It includes persons, institutions, and principles.

Sooner or later, I run out of names. I might come back and add other names as they occur to me, but at this point, I move on.

Next, I start on Column #2, "What happened?" For each name, I think, "Okay, why is that name there?" Just a short point-form summary of the facts, to remind me why the name is on the list. Sometimes it is blank; the name showed up in my list, but I cannot remember what happened. I leave it blank; the "What happened" might show up later.

Now, for each name and "What happened?" entry, I write out, "How It Affected Me." As with Column #3, sometimes I have to leave an entry blank, understanding that I might come back later on in the process. If there is an entry, it is short, often just a few words, like *made me angry, feel shame, feel embarrassed, feel guilty, envious, jealous, afraid, ignited financial fears, made me fearful of my social standing or reputational risk.*

In one of my very few departures from standard Big Book methodology, I have found it more powerful to use my own words, words that come to mind when I think "How did this affect me?"

Finally, the last column — "What was my part?" For this column, the time frame is relevant. For old stuff, what was my part at that time? It might be nothing or everything. And for anything that continues to prey on my mind, *What is my part in hanging on to this today? Why do I not let it go?*

By the time I start the last column, patterns are emerging. Auto-fill on my spreadsheet is starting to pop up more and more frequently because the same words are showing up again and again. Phrases like *I felt entitled; I allowed myself to feel an exaggerated sense of hurt; I was dependent on what they thought; I was overly sensitive; I had puffed myself up and created the situation that created the shame; my expectations were inappropriate; and I was dominated by what people thought of me.*

When completed, I have found patterns and habits that have caused problems. Causes and conditions have been revealed in black and white. I cannot bullshit the paper.

Fifth Step, Redux

Tagged: #spiritual growth, #removing defects, #step 5, #step 6, #step 7

Recently, I relearned the value of Step Five. It releases the power of secrets by talking to another human being. Confession releases and relieves the inner tension caused by secrets. Even secrets that surface from deep down inside.

An event from years before, resurfaced in my mind.

Like a submarine breaking the surface from the depths, it came from a hidden region of my brain. It appeared out of nowhere and presented itself to my conscious awareness. How or why that particular memory came up to the surface is a mystery. There was no apparent trigger but, having reached the surface, it was buoyant and stayed afloat; it persistently itched my conscious awareness.

It wasn't big, or even meaningful, neither to the people involved, nor to me. It was not something that required attention; it was long past. Showing up to make an amend would have seemed odd, to everyone concerned. But it kept grabbing my attention. It was not a continuous presence in my mind, but an itch that I needed to scratch.

At the end of my annual Step Five interview with Father Kevin, my spiritual coach, I shared with him this small itch. It was not part of the general confession and inventory review for that year; it did not seem that important. As we were wrapping up the annual interview, it came to my mind.

I said, "Before we go, I have to tell you something. I've never told anyone. It's not very big or very impressive, but here it is." In less than 50 words, I told him. He paused, holding the door. He said, "Now it has been spoken… good. That is all that needs to be done today."

Immediately I felt relief. I felt better; and once again had affirmed that these Steps work. Not just the first time around, but time and time again.

Don't think about it; just do it.

Acronyms and Word Play

Introduction

My wife and I are investors. In this work, we invent and use acronyms. They summarize experiences and serve as a useful memory aid. I use them in private conversations with my wife and partner to remind us of the lessons we have learned. It helps in a crisis, a quick reminder that this has happened before, frequently enough that we came up with an acronym, so don't be upset, this is just one more time.

For example, many of our investments were ULTI's, Unintended Long-Term Investments. All of our investments included AFLE's: Another Frigging Learning Experience. If the number of zeros involved in the venture increased, the 'F' word changed.

I use acronyms in business and professional meetings, a humorous reminder to make a point.

And I love playing with words. As a lawyer, I know the importance of words. They are the product of our work as lawyers. Whether spoken in court or board meetings, written in contracts or memos, words are the substance and product of the legal profession. Words are dynamic and powerful, but they can be fun as well. Acronyms are like words, they are powerful and dynamic, and we can play around with them.

Turning from my business and personal experience to our 12-Step Program, words are critical. It is all we have to work with. Bill, Dr. Bob, and the founders used words to write a Book that ensured that their message of hope and experience would be applied consistently and successfully. In our shares and speeches, words alone are used. Words are how we communicate with each other and with God.

This chapter draws on my fun with words and affection for acronyms. I hope you enjoy them.

ID the ID

Tagged: #spiritual growth, #inventory, #step 10, #habits, #awareness of god

When I am off the spiritual beam and relying on my own resources and abilities, not trusting in God, not asking Him for directions and not even aware of Him, the most frequent feeling I have is a sense of Impending Doom, ID. What does this feel like? I can only describe it as an unfocused, unattributed sense that something is going to go wrong, and soon.

I develop a deep feeling of ID.

But ID is already an acronym for identification; as in "The police ID'd him as the culprit."

When I have the feeling of impending doom now, I can ID the culprit. I can ID the cause of my ID; it is self-possession and self-centred thinking. It is complete reliance on my resources, my will, my Power, and me.

I can ID the ID, and it is me.

Alcoholic Thinking? GIGO?

Tagged: #attitudes, #feelings, #spiritual growth

In the Rooms of Alcoholics Anonymous, I sometimes hear the expression "alcoholic thinking."

But I wonder, is there anything that can be called alcoholic thought? If I had alcoholic thinking, then my thinking should have changed when I sobered up. That did not happen. But something did happen.

Thinking refers to thought processes like logic, inference, and decision making. These processes did not change when I sobered up and started working the Steps. My thinking did not change. Reasoning and the mental ability to connect actions and consequences, my mental operations and processes, all stayed the same.

What did change, when I stopped drinking and started working the Steps, were the lenses through which I saw the world. These lenses were my perceptions and attitudes. It wasn't my thinking that was flawed. It was the inputs to my thinking that were flawed. My perceptions and attitudes distorted the way that I saw the world.

Alcoholic attitudes like "It's all about me," "I am the most important," "These people are out to get me," and "All that matters here is tha my feelings are hurt" affected my views of reality. Alcoholic perceptions like: "I know what he is thinking," "This is intolerably bad," and "This is unjust" altered my understanding of the world around me. Attitudes and perceptions affected how I saw the world, the inputs to my thinking. This, in turn, defined the outputs: my thoughts, and conclusions.

When I stopped drinking, my ability to logically deduce, inferentially conclude, and other similar mental processes were unchanged. But new attitudes which included: "My Higher Power will help with this," and "The world is unfolding following a Higher Power's will and direction," together with perceptions like "I am not the centre of the universe," and "Others can be helped by this action" affected how I saw the world, the inputs to my thinking. I could see the world more clearly and with truth, as my Higher Power would direct. This, in turn, affected my thought: the outputs.

Instead of my mind following the GIGO rule: "garbage in, garbage out," my mind now follows the law, GIGO, "good in, good out."

At least that has been my experience.

The Meaning of Resentment

Tagged: #spiritual growth, #self will, #resentments, #acronyms, #reacting to the world, #judging in the program

Our Program is life or death. And our Program is made up of words. So the meaning of the words of our Program is a matter of life and death.

Knowing this, I like to keep a dictionary by my side when reading AA material. I like to look up words. Even when I think I know the meaning, I am surprised by errors in my understanding of Program words.

Let's look at resentment, a critical AA word. In the Big Book, it is identified as the number one problem in recovery.

The dictionary definition of resentment is "a feeling of bitter indignation arising from perceived harm or wrong."

Wow.

Let's unpack this dictionary definition. First, it is a feeling, not a fact. Second, the feeling is a sense of indignation, which in turn means anger or annoyance. Third, the source of that feeling is a *perception* of harm or wrong, not *actual* harm or wrong.

That definition surprised me. I wanted to learn more, so I studied the etymology of the word and investigated the prefix 're.' I had always assumed that the prefix 're' was Latin for repeated, meaning that the feelings, the Latin word 'sentir,' were repeated. But I discovered that the prefix 're' has many nuanced and subtle meanings. It includes a sense of repetition, but it also includes additive strengthening like re-inforcement or making something new as in re-newing; and most importantly, to concentrate or focus as in re-fine.

So the meaning of this important word, resentment, the number one killer for alcoholics, is complex. When I thought about my story, these complexities and nuances were significant. Resentments were not merely feelings that were repeated. They were much more than that.

It is worth paying close attention to the meaning of critical words.

A2

Tagged: #acronyms, #ahh 2, #changes

A or *To*.

Let me start this GEM with two grammatical definitions:

'a' — an indefinite article. Example: I need a change.

'to' — a preposition, which could, depending on its use, also be an infinitive. Example: I need to change.

These words are different. They are not synonyms. If you use one word, you are pointed in one direction; if you use the other, you have a completely different goal in mind.

I found that the words *a* and *to* made a difference in my life. When I was drinking, I thought that I needed *a* change. But *a* change never worked. I tried *a* change to my location, *a* change to what I drank, *a* change in my circumstances, lifestyle, and jobs. I tried changes in everything around me, but nothing worked, I still had a drinking problem.

It turns out that I needed *to* change. Without any change in my circumstances, I started working the Steps. This changed me. I needed *to* change my character, *to* change my reactions, *to* change my relationship with a Higher Power. Against all the odds, I stopped drinking.

I needed *to* change, not *a* change.

Now, working on Emotional Sobriety, the same rule applies. My happiness, joy, and freedom are not increasing because of *a* change. Nothing I change in my circumstances or surroundings has a permanent effect on my happiness, joy, or freedom. My happiness, joy, and freedom increase when I strive *to* change.

How to change? Continued work on personal inventories (daily, quarterly, and annual) to reveal patterns and themes in my life that are blocking my spiritual progress: character and moral defects which mature and grow into harmful acts and bad behaviours.

These powerful inventory habits, extended with thoughtful synthesis into the exact nature of the wrongs, are then combined with prayer and meditation, on God and with God as I understood Him, asking Him with humility to remove these defects. This process of identification and removal has increased my happiness, joy, and freedom as I trudge along the road of Happy Destiny.

There is a specific and definite outcome of the processes of the Program — I change. I need *to* change, not *a* change.

This has been my experience and story.

The last stop

Tagged: #fellowship, #love, #program, #unconditional

Recently a speaker reminded me that "AA is the last stop on the railway track to ruin."

There is no next stop. When we came to AA, we were at the end of the tracks. We had reached the final point of desperation. We were at the 'jumping off place.' We had hit the end of the line.

These understandings of that phrase are correct, but there is another understanding of the phrase "AA is the last stop on the railway track to ruin."

To demonstrate, let me share my own story. In my last days of drinking, I was not in trouble. I was in third-year law school, had never been in jail, never charged with any alcohol-related activities; my reputation was still mostly intact. In short, I had many more possible stopping off points on the track to ruin.

I was, in the jargon, a high bottom drunk.

All that I had was a desire to stop drinking. I came to the Rooms, and I was accepted and loved unconditionally, and that is why that Meeting was my last stop. The love and acceptance I received meant that I did not want to get back on the train and go to another stop. It was not the last stop on the railway track. There was more potential ruin ahead, but it was *my* last stop, a loving stop.

The second meaning of "AA is the last stop on the railway track to ruin" refers to the fact that the Rooms are the last stop because newcomers choose to stay, if we love them enough. They may only have the minimum qualification, a slight desire to stop drinking. But that is sufficient if they are invited to stay in a loving and caring manner. If they are welcomed like a long-lost friend.

The second meaning of the last stop is not for the newcomer; it is for the Old-Timers. When we meet a newcomer, we must love them and accept them unconditionally and want them to want to stay, so it becomes the last stop for them.

We create a desire to stop; their first Meeting can become their last stop.

ISM Incredibly Short and Shallow Memory

Tagged: #acronyms, #meditation, #memory, #planning, #step 10, #steps

On Thursday, I went to a men's Meeting in La Jolla. It was a great Meeting, good Fellowship and good shares.

One of the speakers referenced the suffix 'ism.'

He said, "In the Rooms, we often refer to alcoholism as an 'ism' disease. ISM is an acronym for Incredibly Short Memory."

What a great truth. When I was drinking, I could not remember the results of the last drunk, even if it was the night before. But that was just one early manifestation of ISM. I had many more after I had been in the Rooms for a longer time.

Later, when I sobered up and started going to Meetings, but before I began working the Steps, I continued to suffer from ISM. I could not remember the results of my last anger event, temper tantrum, gossip, self-centred sex thinking, or many other harmful behaviours, with sufficient force to stop me from doing it again.

Both before and after AA, I had an ISM. I had an Incredibly Short Memory.

However, with the Program and regular personal inventories followed by constructive amends and actions, I have been able to lengthen my memory. With the habits of inventories and amends, I can now remember the previous time I did something stupid, and because I have had to make amends, I can recall it with enough force to avoid the same behaviours.

Alcoholism is like perfectionism, judgmentalism and absolutism. All of them start with an Incredibly Short Memory. But with continuous inventories, I can improve my memory and defeat the ISM condition.

Abandon or Surrender

Tagged: #abandon, #growth, #step 3, #surrender

My sponsor came up with a great acronym.

NUTS = Not Using The Steps

If I am adrift, not spiritually grounded, then I am NUTS. Not Using The Steps.

When I am Using The Steps, things go well. When my mind is not oriented towards the Steps, I am NUTS.

If you are going to Meetings but seem to be a bit crazy, you might be NUTS.

That is to say, you might be nuts, and the reason might be nuts — you are Not Using The Steps.

Because you are NUTS, you are nuts. Or, you are nuts to NUTS.

We can have great Fellowship in the Program, enjoying the Meetings and coffee sessions and staying sober. However, if you are not baking the Steps into your life, look out.

At least that is my story. For years, I had a great Fellowship and a lousy Program.

Then I started focusing on the Steps, and balance was achieved; life became manageable. Lack of power had been my dilemma and the Fellowship solved it by giving me some potential, but for the additional power to develop character I needed the Steps. I had to work the Program.

So to my sponsor, thanks for the acronym. Thanks too for your supportive and helpful presence throughout my sobriety.

Because You are NUTS, You are Nuts.

Tagged: #spiritual awakening, #spiritual growth, #steps

My sponsor, came up with a great acronym.

N.U.T.S. Not Using The Steps.

If I am adrift, not spiritually grounded, then I am NUTS. Not Using The Steps.

When I am Using The Steps, things go well. When my mind is not oriented towards the Steps, I am NUTS.

So if you are going to meetings but seem to be a bit crazy, you might be NUTS.

That is to say, you might be nuts, and the reason might be nuts - you are Not Using The Steps.

Because you are NUTS, you are nuts. Or, you are nuts to NUTS.

We can have great fellowship in the Program, enjoying the meetings and coffee sessions; and staying sober. However, if you are not baking the steps into your life, look out.

At least that is my story. For years I had a great fellowship and a lousy program.

Then I started focusing on the Steps, and balance was achieved; life became manageable. For lack of power had been my dilemma and the fellowship solved it by giving me some potential, but for the additional power to develop character I needed the Steps, I had to work the Program.

So to my sponsor, thanks for the acronym. Also, thanks too for your supportive and helpful presence throughout my sobriety.

ANDY C

Non-Sequiters — Even When You Don't Want To

Tagged: #program, #spiritual awakening, #steps

Non-sequitur: A conclusion or statement that does not logically follow from the previous statement or proposition. From the Latin "It does not follow."

Our Program is a series of non-sequiturs.

I pointed out to my first sponsor that nowhere in the 12 Steps does it say: "Now we stopped drinking." If the Steps are the solution to my drinking problem, it is curious that they have nothing to say about my drinking. I am never asked to stop drinking. The whole Program is a non-sequitur to the drinking problem.

Of course, I was trying to demonstrate just how bright I was. I wanted him to see what a treasure of a sponsee he had.

He paused, then gave me an answer, which at the time appeared to be another non-sequitur. He told me he was going to pick me up in 20 minutes because we had a 12-Step call.

I demanded to know what that had to do with my observation about the Steps and my drinking. He just replied, "20 minutes. Be out in front of your building." He did not answer my question or even comment on my insight. It was as if he ignored what I had to say. He did that a lot.

But going on that 12-Step call kept me from drinking. It may have seemed like a non-sequitur, but it was right on point.

Our Program answers do not seem to follow the question: *How do I stop drinking?*

But it works. It is doing actions even though I don't see their connection to the problems.

143

Moral inventories — didn't want to do them, but did them anyway.

Personal inventories — didn't like them, but did them anyway.

12-Step calls — What does any of this have to do with my allergic reaction to alcohol and my inability to remember the last drunk with sufficient force to prevent me from doing it again?

I didn't know, but I did it anyway.

There are still so many things in this Program that I don't understand and cannot connect to drinking. In my mind, so much of what we do appears to be a non-sequitur.

But I have learned that there is a connection between these actions and sobriety. My sponsor picked me up, and we made a 12-Step call. I never looked back. He answered my question with a 12-Step action.

Now Here — Nowhere

Tagged: #spiritual growth, #God as I understood Him, #self-centered, #growing up, #attitudes

Vital wordplay.

Have you noticed that if you are in the moment, "Now Here," then you are somewhere? Life has meaning. But if you bang those words together you are NowHere, nowhere, and life has no meaning; your connection to a Higher Power is lost and Nowhere to be found.

That little space between Now and Here is essential.

In London, England, on the subway platforms, you see signs that warn you to "Mind the gap." And the conductors shout, "Mind the gap." They mean the gap between the trains and the platform. Because if you ignore the gap, the subway train will crush you.

In the Rooms, we could have signs that say, "Mind the gap." If you ignore the gap between Now and Here, life will crush you.

Mind the Gap between Now and Here.

EGO — Edging God Out

Tagged: #inventory, #spiritual awakening, #spiritual growth

Every morning, I pray and meditate. As I arise from my knees, my conscious contact with God could be rated at a ten out of ten. But a mere 30 minutes later, if I stopped and thought about it, my conscious contact with God rating would be down to seven out of ten. By eleven o'clock, my conscious awareness rating is down to two or three out of ten and declining. By 1:00 pm, I am in full control of my life, and my conscious contact rating is zero.

Nothing dramatic will have happened, just a series of thoughts and decisions that can be summarized as, "Don't worry God, I've got this;" I gently edge God out of my consciousness.

I am like the practising alcoholic who swears off alcohol at 9:00 am, develops a thirst by noon, and at 4:00 pm concludes that "Tomorrow will be an excellent day to quit." It just seems to happen. Nothing dramatic, not a decision. I am just edging towards the booze, edging out of sobriety.

In the same way, I don't decide to release God from my consciousness; I Edge Him Out.

I don't tell God to "Get lost." I don't say, "That's it; I am terminating my conscious contact with You." Rather a separation from God creeps up on me. I Edge God Out rather than order Him out.

I need a reminder to get back to a higher conscious contact with God. I have found a technology solution, a way to combat this process of EGO, Edging God Out.

The solution for me is a series of alarms on my phone. I have programmed my phone with alarms that go off at the same time every day. I have five during the day. Each alarm is silent, with only a 'screen flash' alert. I label the alarms with short, concise messages. The label for each alarm is a message to remind me to be consciously aware of God, like *God is here; God is in this; God loves you; God has a will for you; God is in charge.*

Five times a day, my phone alerts me, and when I pay attention, it stops the unconscious process of Edging God Out — EGO.

Maybe I should have a second acronym. Daily Alarm Technology Solution — DATS. DATS prevents EGO.

EGO? DATS all, folks!

Sobriety is not Circumstantial

Tagged: #action, #circumstances, #program, #steps

Recently, I attended the monthly Simon House Graduation and Birthday Meeting in Calgary. It's a terrific evening — full of energy and hope.

Graduates and residents from prior years who are celebrating birthdays gave short 'shares.' One caught my ear: "Sobriety is not circumstantial."

True, so true. True for both my alcoholism and my sobriety.

My alcoholism was not circumstantial. It didn't depend on my circumstances. I could and would drink anywhere, anytime, for any reason. I would just drink; it always seemed like the natural thing to do.

In my early sobriety, I did not stop drinking because of my circumstances. Nothing in my circumstances changed. I changed because of the Fellowship and the Program, persistently applied to my life.

I can see that there is nothing circumstantial about my spiritual growth and serenity. The changes are all on the inside, not the outside. They are the result of enjoying spiritual awakenings which are the direct result of the persistent application of the Steps to all areas of my life.

In my experience, my drinking was not circumstantial, and my growth in sobriety is not circumstantial. It is internal, a persistent and determined effort to maintain my spiritual condition.

My sobriety has required effort, persistence, and actions.

We might need some new words to include these concepts, words like *effort-itial* and *persistent-itial.*

ANDY C

A Parting GEM

Unconditional Love

Tagged: #spiritual growth, #love, #growing up, #small things,
#growth, #emotional sobriety, #conscious awareness, #self-centered,
#wives, #hard work, #discipline

I observe the unconditional love we show newcomers to the Program.

They come in nervously, with apprehension and fear. They identify themselves. They become the centre of the Meeting. We love them. We circulate newcomer packages, and every share starts with "Welcome to the newcomer; we all had our first Meeting." Meeting topics suddenly include the first Step.

If they falter, we pick them up. If they turn on us, we forgive them. If they abandon us and go back to drinking, we move on. If they come back, we welcome them again. They can do no wrong that we cannot forgive. They cannot disappoint us. We have no expectations that can be frustrated. We welcome them and greet them at the door with a smile and a handshake (and maybe a hug).

Sponsees get the same unconditional love: If they call, we are only interested in how we can help. We listen with patience, kindness, and understanding.

Unconditional love.

What if I could apply these rules of conduct, behaviour, and attitude to others outside of the Program? What if I could practise these principles in all my affairs?

What if I could deal with all people as if they were newcomers or sponsees?[12] What if we could forgive them and show unconditional patience and love?

What if we could meet and tolerate, with love: Fellow workers who take our ideas and make us look bad? Employers who mistreat us with cross words and criticisms? Clients who fail to praise us? Spouses who irritate and criticize us? Even in the Rooms, alcoholics who irritate us and, of course, the inevitable Meeting drones? What if we could treat them all like newcomers and sponsees?

Who knows what our lives would be like? For me, I don't know yet; I have not achieved that level of spiritual growth. But I can hope, can't I?

---

[12] An old sponsor of mine used to tell me a variation of this rule. He saw how assiduously I served my clients. He said, "You should treat your wife as well as you would new clients." New clients did no wrong, could not be criticized, and were served with unquestioned enthusiasm. Could I treat my spouse that way?

Bibliography

The Best of Bill, by AA Grapevine

The Big Book of Alcoholics Anonymous Paperback, by Dr. Bob Smith, Bill Wilson [The First and Second Editions of the Big Book, Alcoholics Anonymous, are in the public domain in the United States only. The Third and Fourth Editions remain copyright protected worldwide, including the United States.]

Dr. Bob and the Good Oldtimers, by Alcoholics Anonymous

Happy, Joyous & Free: The Lighter Side of Sobriety, by AA Grapevine

Not God: A History of Alcoholics Anonymous, by Ernest Kurtz

Twelve Steps and Twelve Traditions, by Anonymous

Books that have meant a lot to me

AA Supplied Literature
>The Big Book
Twelve Steps and Twelve Traditions
Pass It On
Dr Bob and the Good Old Timers

Books that the founders read (the Recovery Bible)
>The Greatest Thing in the World
The Will to Believe
Varieties of Religious Experiences
Sermon on the Mount
A Design for Living
The Greatest Thing in the World
1st Corinthians
The Book of James
The Peabody book

Books about drinking alcoholically
>My Name is Bill W. (The book and the movie)
The Lost Weekend (The book and the movie)

Modern AA Underground
>The Road Less Traveled

Books I have learned from
>The Akron Genesis of AA
The Interior Castle
Father Ed Dowling, Bill Wilson's Sponsor
The Power of Your Subconscious Mind
How to Live Without Worry

You can get Andy C's GEMS in your email
by subscribing at:

https://the4thdimension.ca/subscribe/

Biography

Andy C. has captured large elements of his sobriety with this book. Many of the lessons portrayed in the stories are from his experiences and observations as a successful lawyer, social leader and parent.

He was born in small town Ontario, Canada. He sobered up in his third year of law school, November 3, 1977. He graduated from Lakehead University with a Commerce and Finance Degree and then completed a Law Degree at the University of Toronto. He moved to Calgary. He married his wife Doreen and they have two children.

For Andy, not drinking was a first spiritual awakening. He's been blessed with subsequent spiritual awakenings as the result of the practice of the program of Alcoholics Anonymous and good sponsorship.

Andy is active in service work in AA, and was been instrumental in the foundation and ongoing growth of Simon House in Calgary. He was also a leader in the Lawyers' Assist Program of Alberta, assisting lawyers in crisis often with booze and alcohol. Andy is involved in prodigious 12-step work. He is sponsored and sponsors others, and has a Home Group.

Index

A

abandon · 39, 146
acceptance · 21
acronyms · 138, 140, 144
action · 154
agnostics · 27, 71
ahh 2 · 140
alarms · 29
amends · 48
anger · 25, 48, 98, 102
annual · 112, 120, 128
appearances · 60
attitudes · 136, 151
awareness · 29, 44, 53,
    71, 74, 76, 104, 135

B

businessman on the
    beach · 39

C

changes · 54, 74, 140
checklist · 41, 50, 77
circumstances · 154
coincidence · 76
complications · 107
conscious awareness · 44,
    71, 100, 156

D

daily checklist · 126
denial · 39
dependency on the
    opinion of others · 44,
    122
discipline · 41, 71, 114,
    116, 118, 122, 124, 156

E

emotional sobriety · 23,
    33, 36, 44, 71, 100, 112,
    156

F

faith · 93
fear · 39, 107
feelings · 111, 136
fellowship · 142
forgiveness · 89
freedom · 89

G

God as I understood
    Him · 29, 43, 93, 102,
    151
good and evil · 19
growing up · 25, 44, 46,
    82, 112, 151, 156

growth · 39, 98, 100, 146, 156

H

habits · 19, 41, 44, 71, 114, 116, 118, 120, 122, 124, 126, 135
hard work · 156
house building · 65

I

in the moment · 58, 71, 95
inventory · 36, 52, 62, 102, 111, 112, 114, 116, 118, 120, 122, 124, 128, 135, 152

J

judging in the program · 27, 138

L

lack of power · 54
love · 17, 142, 156

M

maintenance · 74
measurement of results · 48
meditation · 29, 53, 56, 71, 84, 144
meetings · 76

memory · 144
morning checklist · 50, 126
morning meditation · 50, 71, 126

N

naming defects · 114
need for praise · 122
nowhere · 25

P

planning · 144
prayer · 48, 71
present · 58, 95
pride · 98
program · 17, 46, 87, 142, 149, 154
pushing buttons · 54

R

reacting to the world · 54, 138
removing defects · 31, 116, 118, 130
resentments · 89, 138
restless irritable and discontented · 93

S

self-centered · 44, 97, 98, 105, 112, 151, 156
serenity · 21
small things · 122, 156

spiritual awakening · 27, 33, 36, 39, 41, 43, 46, 48, 60, 67, 69, 74, 79, 93, 100, 102, 120, 124, 147, 149, 152

spiritual experiences · 93, 120

spiritual growth · 19, 23, 25, 27, 29, 31, 33, 36, 41, 53, 54, 56, 60, 62, 65, 67, 71, 76, 77, 79, 84, 89, 100, 112, 120, 130, 135, 136, 138, 147, 151, 152, 156

steps · 23, 46, 65, 67, 69, 71, 77, 79, 82, 84, 87, 107, 120, 126, 144, 147, 149, 154

   step 10 · 27, 36, 41, 52, 54, 104, 112, 114, 116, 118, 120, 128, 135, 144

   step 11 · 29, 50, 71, 84, 100, 104

   step 12 · 23, 60, 69

   step 2 · 33, 79

   step 3 · 43, 60, 77, 146

   step 4 · 89, 122, 124, 128

   step 5 · 102, 105, 112, 116, 118, 130

   step 6 · 31, 130

   step 7 · 31, 130

   step 9 · 87

stories · 48

subsequent awakenings · 36, 114

surrender · 71, 146

T

thinking · 17

tools of the program · 44, 67, 71

U

unconditional · 17, 142

W

Wilson, Bill · 84

wives · 17, 156

working the steps · 112, 114, 116, 118, 126

CPSIA information can be obtained
at www.ICGtesting.com
Printed in the USA
LVHW032348160919
631244LV00006B/14/P

9 781999 240707